Natural Healing
With
Water, Herbs &
Sunlight

by Maureen O'Rourke

INTRODUCTION

Water is the foundation of life on planet earth. Water nurtures and soothes, cleanses and purifies, refreshes, revitalizes and renews the body and the spirit.

Consider the simple shower. Whether you are showering at the beginning of the day, as a transition to a new activity during the day, or rinsing off in the evening, you certainly have experienced the transformational power of water. Besides washing off the physical sweat of life's activities, water clears away mental and emotional residues as well. You feel like a new person, ready to face the next adventure.

Add to this basic understanding a purposeful control of temperature and form. Enhance it with the addition of herbs or plant extracts. Apply it to any number of situations where the soothing, cleansing and revitalizing influences of water (as ice, liquid, or vapors) would be needed and appreciated.

As typical humans in this modern society, we get caught up in the demands of daily life, and too often forget that we have such a powerful healing tool so easily within reach. Discover the abundance of opportunities to use water as a supportive tool in your everyday life. Place yourself under the influence of a strong jet of water, a hot infusion, a cold plunge, an herbal wrap, or whatever inspires you. Shake loose the entrapments of daily life and rinse away the layer of tension used to hold onto this baggage.

As hydrotherapy is included in the movement toward the use of adjunct therapies in the treatment of modern ills and injuries, it is enjoying a comeback into the curricula in schools of massage therapy, physical therapy, athletic training, nursing, and other training institutions. The use of water as a therapeutic medium requires a good understanding of the physiological effects occurring in the body, as well as the most efficient methods for administering the treatments. It is equally important that the training include a practical component, which not only gives student therapists an experience of applying the techniques, but also gives them an opportunity to experience the treatments themselves.

Maureen O'Rourke artfully presents a simplified view of the complex physiology of the body in relationship to the effects of hydrotherapeutic applications. She has laid out a logical course of study into this fascinating modality in a clear, easy-to-follow manual. Her inclusion of herbs and heliotherapy, in addition to the water treatments, creates a well-rounded approach to this body of knowledge.

Throughout her text, Ms. O'Rourke weaves the use of water, herbs, and light into the broader fabric of health care. By providing the necessary understanding of indications and contraindications for various treatments, she gives a perspective into its proper use in relationship with other aspects of therapeutic intervention. Here's hoping that having a resource as concise and easy to follow as this book will inspire the use of hydrotherapy in more professional health-care practices, and in the personal regimens of our daily lives.

Iris Burman
Founder; Director
Educating Hands School of Massage Therapy
Miami, Florida

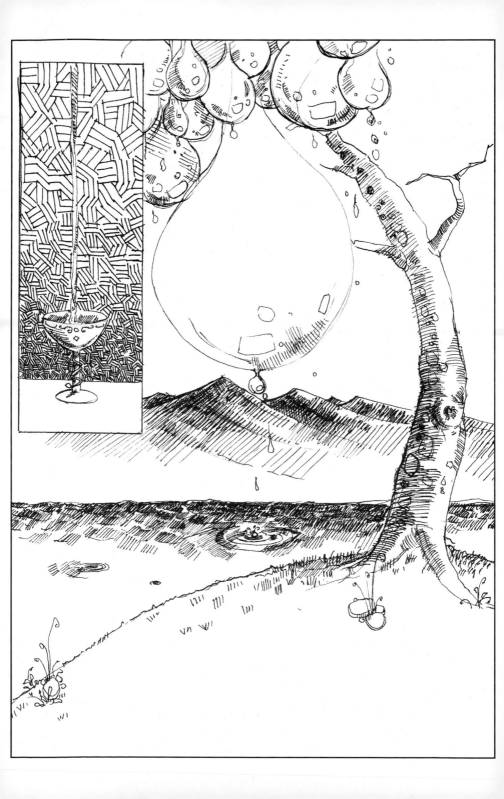

HYDROTHERAPY - NATURAL HEALING WITH WATER

A Brief History of Hydrotherapy

Humankind has long recognized that water does more than simply relieve thirst. Water is the oldest and most universal of all healers, not only used for drinking, but in external applications as well. Its accessibility, ease of application using simple and inexpensive tools, and its ability to absorb and conduct large quantities of heat make water a very versatile healing agent.

Since 3,000 BC, the era of the Egyptian physician **Aesculapius,** we find the concepts of water and healing joined: the Ancient Greeks who lived in later eras considered Aesculapius a god, representing him with a serpent, which is a symbol of living water and our current symbol for the healing arts. His daughter **Hygeia** - origin of the word hygiene, our term for healthful cleansing - was shown with a serpent on her wrist, drinking water from a cup. Pictures found in ancient **Egyptian** tombs show preparations for bathing in their sacred river, the Nile. **Ancient Hebrews, Persians, Babylonians and Assyrians** used water in the treatment of disease; in an ancient **Chinese** text, a physician prescribed ice water treatments followed by wrapping in a sheet (the original wet sheet wrap)! Citizens of the Greek city-state **Sparta** were required to take cold baths to harden the body and stimulate metabolism. Elsewhere around the world, we find traditional water treatments being handed down throughout the generations - the **Finnish** dry sauna followed by a roll in the snow, the **Japanese** steam baths, **American Indian** sweat lodges and mineral water springs baths, and purification by water baptism noted in the **Bible**, as well as in other religious teachings. The emperor Charlemagne is said to have held court while relaxing in a huge warm bath. Public vapor baths were numerous in Paris in 1600 A D, often connected with barber shops, where the red and white striped barber poles outside these establishments indicated that bleeding treatments for various diseases were also performed.

The Greek physician **Hippocrates**, the "Father of Modern Medicine," in 500 BC used baths and hot fomentations to heal his patients. He obviously understood the physiological effects on the body of water at varying temperatures, including the idea that cold baths should be of short duration, accompanied by friction treatments, so as not to drain the body's energy supplies. He documented the phenomenon of **reaction**, the body's protective response to temperatures above or below body norms, in noting that a short cold bath encourages the body to quickly recuperate its heat and remain warm, while a hot bath produces the opposite effect.

Aesclepiades, another Greek physician (about 91 BC), is credited with making quite a "splash" in Rome by introducing Greek healing methods, including hydrotherapy, massage and exercise. Aesclepiades employed hot and cold baths, douches, compresses, fomentations, and many other forms of hydrotherapy. The first public baths in ancient **Rome** were built in 312 BC, using only cold water. Eventually these became "thermae," adapted to the use of warm water as well, and were developed over time to accommodate up to 10,000 bathers daily. And, by AD 302, the newly-completed baths of Diocletian could hold up to 1,000 bathers at one time! Typical **thermae** had several different chambers, including a dressing room, a chamber for anointing the body with oil, an area for athletic games to be played, two heated chambers, one dry and one steam (where curved metal tools, called stirgils, were used to scrape off sweat and dirt, since soap did not yet exist), and a warm bath followed by a cold one. The imperial physician Galen prescribed cold water therapy for various ills of the body, and healing in Rome during five centuries in this era was almost totally confined to the public baths, according to the historian Pliny.

During the **Dark Ages** in England and Europe, water treatments and bathing fell into disrepute. In the seventeenth century, perfumes replaced baths, as nudity was considered a sin. Queen Isabella of Spain is said to have taken two baths in her lifetime - at birth and marriage - and this was considered normal and proper at that time! (Arabic physicians, including **Avicenna,** the "Arab Prince of Doctors," kept alive the traditions of water therapy which might otherwise have been lost.) A giant of seventeenth century English medicine, **Dr. Thomas Sydenham**, when writing on treatment of fevers, actually apologized for recommending the use of hydrotherapy treatments as being preferable to the current practice of "bleeding out the bad humors" in the treatment of fevers. His fears of destroying his practice and reputation were probably well-founded, knowing as we do how slowly people adapt to "new" ideas. Despite the detractors, however, Sydenham was praised after his death, called by some the "English Hippocrates" or the "Father of English Medicine."

Early in the nineteenth century, a poor Silesian peasant named **Vincent Preissnitz** (1799-1852) popularized the use of cold water for curative measures. As a boy on his father's farm he noticed that folk remedies using cold water were very effective in healing the farm animals' sprains and bruises. At the age of seventeen, when he suffered a severe injury to his chest accompanied by broken ribs, the doctors offered him no hope of a cure. Preissnitz experimented with cold towels and cold drinking water, ultimately healing himself successfully. As word of his self-cure got around, he began treating friends and neighbors, often alternating sweating treatments with the cold water applications. Among those who heard of Preissnitz' cures was a German named **Sebastian Kneipp** (1821-1897), who, because he was afflicted with consumption (tuberculosis) was advised he could never enter the priesthood. Experimenting with modified diet, cold water and sweating treatments such as body wraps and baths, he cured himself and realized his dream of becoming a priest. "Father" Kneipp then began treating his parishioners, using trial and error methods to modify

Preissnitz' hydrotherapy treatments to make them less severe. Kneipp's ideas were spread rapidly throughout the world through his writings - notably Meine Wasserkur ("My Water Cure" - published in 1886), and today in Germany we find many spas (Kurhause), with physicians on staff, incorporating the Kneipp System. A **Kneipp Kur** (course) includes treatments based on five fundamental principles: 1. hydrotherapy (thermal and mechanical water applications and baths), 2. kinesiotherapy (exercise, movement and massage), 3. phytotherapy (natural herbal medicinal remedies, oils, teas, and juices), 4. nutrition (well-balanced, tasty, digestible, and diversified diets), and 5. regulative therapy (mental, emotional, rhythmic, and cultural life patterns).

During this same time period, the Hungarian physician **Ignaz Phillip Semmelweiss** was encountering great controversy over his ideas. He postulated that the current practice of the day, in which doctors went directly from the autopsy room to deliver babies, was a major cause of "childbed fever." He tried to get those physicians to wash their hands between treatments to prevent infection, but was met with such resistance that it undermined his health and spirit. He was taken to a mental hospital in 1865, where ironically he died of sepsis, the blood infection he had spent most of his life trying to eradicate.

Yet also during the nineteenth century, noted European universities offered courses taught by such respected figures as **Wilhelm Winternitz** (1834-1912), professor of hydrotherapy at the University of Vienna and a famed neurologist. As a result of seeing the work of Preissnitz and others, Winternitz wrote over 200 articles and books scientifically documenting the physiological effects of water treatments on the body. He studied in particular those effects happening through the nervous system. Winternitz became a mentor of the Americans Dr. John Harvey Kellogg and **Dr. Simon Baruch**. Baruch, who later worked for legislation in America to regulate hydrotherapy and eliminate quackery, became professor of hydrotherapy at the College of Physicians and Surgeons at Columbia University.

John Harvey Kellogg (1852-1943) was instrumental in spreading European developments in hydrotherapy and hygiene across the Atlantic Ocean. He introduced spas to America when he established his Battle Creek Sanitarium in Michigan. Here treatment methods encompassed the best aspects of the healing arts. Healthful diet modifications (he touted corn flakes & milk as a healthy alternative to artery-clogging ham & eggs breakfasts), hydrotherapy, and spinal manipulation were used alongside current scientific medical procedures of the time, which included some surgery and drug therapy. He achieved outstanding results with this combination, almost without harmful side effects, in treating patients with pneumonia, nephritis, serious infections, musculoskeletal pain, and many other kinds of "dis-eases" of the body. Kellogg's book Rational Hydrotherapy, published in 1901, is still today the definitive text on water

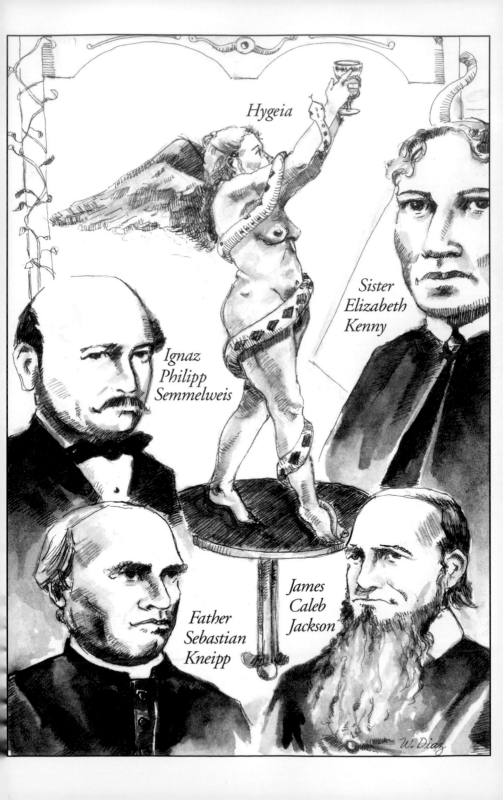

Hygeia

Sister
Elizabeth
Kenny

Ignaz
Philipp
Semmelweis

Father
Sebastian
Kneipp

James
Caleb
Jackson

W. Diaz

therapy, as a result of his thorough development and documentation of techniques, and his exhaustive historical research. It has done much to put the subject of hydrotherapy on a scientific basis.

Another influential American, **James Caleb Jackson** (1814-1895) treated the sick at "Our Home on the Hillside" in Dansville, NY, using no drugs (not even herbs or homeopathic medicines). In his How to Treat the Sick Without Medicine (1874), Jackson outlined his "True Materia Medica," including 1) Air, 2) Simple food, 3) Water, 4) Sunlight, 5) Dress, 6) Exercise, 7) Sleep, 8) Rest, 9) Social influences, and 10) Mental and moral influences.

In Australia, **Sister Elizabeth Kenny** (1886-1952) was experimenting with a novel treatment for poliomyelitis. As a teenager, she studied muscular structure and function in depth in order to help her sickly younger brother, who ultimately became the strongest man in the Australian army. In 1911, at the age of twenty-five, Nurse Kenny was left to care for several cases of infantile paralysis by a doctor who had cabled her that there was "no known treatment" for the disease. The prevailing opinion was that normal strength muscles were overwhelming weakened and wasting antagonistic muscles. The splints and casts that were commonly used to prevent too much malformation were not very successful in relieving either pain or disability: paralysis was assumed to be the unavoidable outcome. Kenny's analysis of polio was that it was a problem where powerful muscle spasms were overwhelming the normal strength of the muscles on the other side of the joint (antagonists). Thus, she used hot fomentations to relax the tight muscles and pool exercises to re-educate the muscles to regain normal function and relieve pain. Her very successful treatments, which she labeled **"heat and motion"** were born out of her desire to ease the children's pain from the contractures. Treatment with hot packs and exercise in a pool, where buoyancy relieves stress on the joints, are both commonly used modalities today, for a wide variety of diseases and musculoskeletal injuries.

Unfortunately, with the advent of many scientific discoveries in the field of allopathic medicine in the United States, hydrotherapeutic procedures fell into disuse. Doctors and nurses, whose previous training included many of these treatments, spent more time studying uses of "miracle" drugs and surgery to heal their patients. Our whole medical system changed to accommodate these new treatments, and medical practitioners dealing with hospital rooms full of needy patients couldn't supply the often time-intensive and labor-intensive hydrotherapy treatments. Negative side effects of drug and surgery treatments have come to light with the passage of time, however, and many people are rediscovering water therapies in their search for affordable health care that won't lead to further complications. Pool therapy exercises used in rehabilitation of athletic injuries, sitz baths to relieve hemorrhoids or prostatitis, and relaxation in a warm bath prior to childbirth to shorten the duration and lessen the pain of labor, are but a few examples of current hydrotherapy treatments. The mindset exemplified by the doctor's cliché phrase "take two aspirins and call me in the morning" is so ingrained, though, that it will take some time before we can make prevention of disease our goal, and truly re-take control of our health through the use of natural healing methods.

The Importance of Water

Water, the most common chemical compound on earth, can be a uniquely effective medicine, healing in the way all true healers do - by stimulating the body's natural immune system to heal itself. We know that drinking water is vital to life - after all, haven't scientists told us that our bodies consist of approximately 60-70% water, which must be continually replenished to maintain health? We have negative feedback mechanisms that allow us to retain extra water in cases of dehydration in order to maintain normal body functions. Our cells and tissues are bathed in this "ocean" of body fluids. It surrounds our brain, circulates through our veins and arteries, helps to digest our food, and fills all of our cells. All of the chemical reactions which make up metabolism - repairing and replacing cells as well as breaking down the food we eat to create energy to think and move - happen in this "body ocean." Interestingly enough, this internal ocean has a very similar chemical makeup to the earth's oceans, which make up approximately 70% of the earth's surface. Included are the major electrolytes sodium, chlorine, bicarbonate, potassium, magnesium, and phosphate. Electrolytes are substances capable of conducting electrical currents when they're found in a solution - dissolved in water, for example. They are the prerequisites necessary for the function of "living matter," in our muscle contractions and nerve impulses. We know we can't survive more than a few days without water. Our Darwinian heritage tells us that the simplest life forms began in the oceans, only crawling upon the land as they evolved. Their systems became complex enough to allow separation from "Mother Ocean," because they developed their own "ocean within."

The earth, and all living things growing upon it, are continually recycling this vital compound. Water evaporates from oceans, lakes and rivers as the sun heats it, wind carries this moisture-laden air to form clouds, and then cooler temperatures cause condensation of these vapors to a liquid or even a solid form as rain, snow, or hail. This water or melting ice then refills those bodies of water. Living creatures drink from the lakes, or ingest water as a part of foods such as fruits, vegetables, grains and meats. It fills all our cells, and is used to dilute and digest foods, move nutrients through the body in the bloodstream, excrete toxins and waste products as urine or feces, cool the body in the form of evaporating perspiration, or moisten the air we breathe. And those perspirations, excretions, urines, tears and moist exhalations of breath return the water to ground water and clouds to continue the cycle.

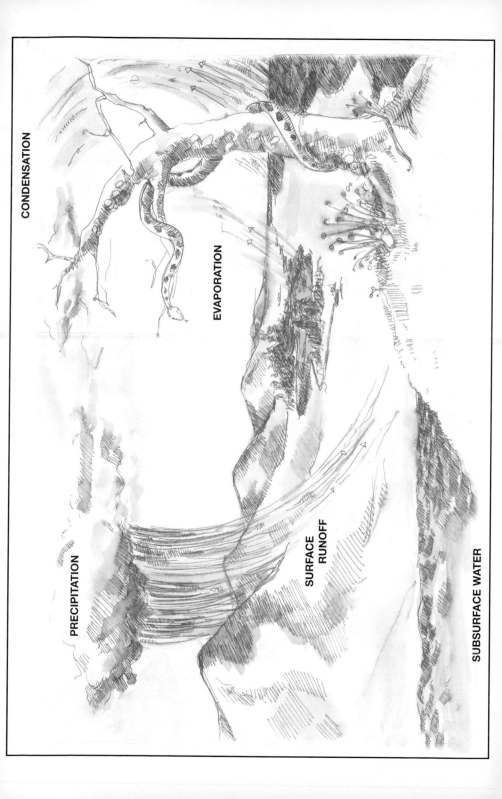

Water (H_2O) Internally . . . . How Important Is It?

Water:

- Makes up **60-70% total body weight**
- Is key in **maintaining endurance and energy levels**
- Is vital for **heat regulation** (thermal homeostasis)
- Oddly enough, drinking water is the best way to **overcome water retention**
- Helps maintain proper **muscle and skin tone** and helps **prevent wrinkles**
- Prevents and **relieves constipation**; is necessary to **digest and process food**

We lose water:

- **2 cups per day** thru **respiration** - more with exercise, dry environment
- **2 cups per day** thru **perspiration** - more with exercise, hot environment
- **6 cups per day** as excretions from **intestines and kidneys**
- Varying amounts: reproductive **secretions, bleeding, vomiting, tears**
- Use 1cc water per calorie ingested to process nutrients and eliminate wastes -
    eating 2,000 calories requires 8½ cups water to process the food
- Thru **coffee, cola, and alcohol consumption; diuretics; medications**

We gain water:

- **3 ½ cups from food** ingested
- **½ cup** formed thru body's **metabolism**
- **We need to drink 6+ cups per day** to function well

Signs of inadequate intake of water:

- **Dark yellow urine,** kidney stones, urinary tract infections
- **Dry mouth,** dry lips, **cold sores** in susceptible people
- **Dehydration** - not always the best indicator, however
- **Constipation, nausea, vomiting**
- **Fatigue, muscle soreness, joint pain**
- **Wrinkles**, dry skin, poor skin tone
- **Overheating** body
- **Swollen feet, legs, hands, face**
- **Dizziness and changes in blood pressure**
- **Disorientation, apathy, depression, aggression**
- **Damage to central nervous system, kidney, liver**
- **Overweight due to water retention**

Temperature and Heat Transfer

The three states of water, as a **gas, liquid, or solid**, exist within a very narrow temperature range: on the Celsius scale, at the **freezing point of 0°** **(32°F)** water becomes ice, and above the **boiling point of 100° (212°F)** it turns into a vapor. This makes it very easy to make applications above and below body temperature to obtain a therapeutic physiological effect. In a phenomenon known as the **latent heat of vaporization,** 540 calories of heat per gram are required to change water to steam. Because of this, the evaporation of water or perspiration has a cooling effect on the body. Conversely, vapor condensing back to a liquid state releases 540 calories, making it clear why steam escaping from an overheated car radiator, for example, can condense on the skin and cause dangerous burns. A similar effect happens when water is frozen into ice. The **latent heat of fusion** releases 80 calories of heat per gram to make ice very useful in refrigeration. And due to that same effect, 80 calories of heat are required to melt a gram of ice, making it very effective at cooling us off.

Because of water's ability to absorb and conduct large quantities of heat, and its ready accessibility, it has been taken as the standard for measuring **specific heat**. It takes 1 calorie of heat to raise 1 gram of water 1°C, so the specific heat of water is "1." We can compare this to air, wood, or cloth, with specific heat values of less than "1" and which conduct heat very poorly; and certain metals such as silver or mercury, at specific heat values higher than "1," which conduct heat extremely well. As an example, because water has 27 times greater capacity to conduct heat than air does, we can briefly walk outside in 32°F weather with our skin bare without feeling too chilled, but if we were to submerge ourselves in a tub of water at that temperature, we would immediately gasp at the shock as the cold water quickly begins to absorb our body heat!

When we refer to "hot" and "cold" in hydrotherapy, we are relating it to normal body temperature. **37°C or 98.6°F is a normal oral body temperature**, although we know that we have a certain range of normal above or below these figures. Body temperature is related to metabolism, or the ability of organisms to break down and assimilate food or energy at a chemical level, and use it to perform functions vital to life, such as waste removal, growth, repair of injured tissues, and movement. The **basal metabolic rate (BMR)**, which can be defined as the energy required to keep a resting body alive, is the number of calories burned per body surface area per hour. It is measured when a person is awake, but resting, and hasn't eaten in 12 hours, and includes the energy requirements for heartbeat, muscle tone, growth, and other basic cell activities. Many mechanisms can alter our BMR. A fever increases it 7% for each degree of increase in body temperature, and pregnancy or physical exercise will also raise our metabolic rate and thus our temperature. Resting or fasting will slow the BMR, conserving energy when it is not needed or not available.

Water Temperature Ranges:

Boiling	212°F	100° C
Dangerously Hot Above	125° F	Above 50° C
Painfully Hot	110- 120° F	42.8- 46° C
Very Hot	104- 110° F	40- 42.8° C
Hot	100- 104° F	38- 40° C
Warm	92- 100° F	34- 38° C
Oral temperature	98.6° F	37° C
Neutral	94- 97° F	34.4- 37° C
Skin temperature	92°F	34°C
Tepid	80- 92° F	27- 34° C
Cool	70- 80° F	21- 27° C
Cold	55- 70° F	3- 21° C
Very Cold	32- 55° F	0- 13° C
Freezing	32° F	0° C

Body temperature is maintained by balancing heat lost against heat gained. We must understand the different ways in which heat can be exchanged with the environment. **Conduction** is an exchange of heat by direct contact of a heated substance with another substance. This is the manner in which a heating pad or an ice pack is effective, and is the method most often used in hydrotherapy. **Convection** is a method by which heat is transferred by moving currents of heated liquid or gas, as in a convection oven or an old-fashioned room radiator. In **conversion**, no heat is applied externally, but is generated within the substance by passing some form of energy through it, such as heating wires by passing electricity through them or using an ultrasound machine to generate sound vibrations in muscles to increase metabolism and warm the tissues. Our bodies lose heat by **evaporation** of water from the skin surface, which takes heat with it. **Radiation** is the giving off of heat as infrared radiation, a type of electromagnetic radiation, which we feel as warmth from the sun or from wood burning in a fire.

Seventy percent of heat loss from the body at room temperature is accomplished via conduction, convection and radiation, twenty-seven percent is lost as result of evaporation of perspiration and moist exhalations, with excretions and heating of inspired air accounting for the balance. As the environmental temperature rises and comes closer to body temperature, however, heat loss is more and more a function of evaporation of perspiration. We must note, though, that if the outside environment is very humid, the water will not evaporate very efficiently since the air is already saturated with water vapor, making evaporation an unreliable heat-dissipating mechanism in humid weather. We also find it harder to breathe in a very humid environment, since very moist air makes the exchange of oxygen gas from the air with carbon dioxide gas in our lungs very difficult.

Homeostasis - Maintaining Balance in our Bodies

Even though we consider healing to be an art requiring creative thinking and sensitivity, it is necessary to be able to predict the probable outcome of a treatment for it to be effective. To accomplish this with hydrotherapy, we must have a basic understanding of the anatomy and physiology of the body, and an understanding of the effects that heat or cold applications will have upon the different body systems.   Basic to this understanding is the concept of **homeostasis,** a Greek term referring to an optimum state of equilibrium, or balance within our bodies. This is a narrow range in the cells' fluid environment with regard to volume, temperature and chemical content, where a cell or organism can function normally to maintain and support life. Many factors can affect this environment, such as seasonal and environmental temperature changes, atmospheric pressure, sunlight or other radiation, rainfall, clothing, food and water supply, and emotions or social conditions. Our bodies thus require certain mechanisms, **negative feedback loops,** in which any deviation from normal is resisted, to maintain the balance.

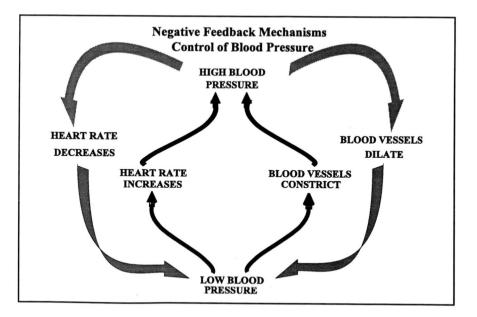

An example of one of these balancing systems can be seen in the maintenance of normal blood pressure and volume. An increase in blood pressure is detected by pressure-sensitive nerve endings in certain arteries, which send signals to the brain. The brain then initiates a sequence of events, including a decrease in heart rate and an increase in the diameter of the blood vessels (relaxing the sphincter muscles controlling capillary blood flow), thus lowering resistance to the flow of blood by increasing the total volume area. The blood spreads out in these vessels, effecting a lowered blood pressure. The sensation of a decrease in blood pressure would have the opposite effect. The blood vessels would be constricted and the heart rate increased to allow the pressure to be raised back to normal.

Another negative feedback example relates to carbon dioxide levels, which help regulate the pH levels and chemical content of the blood. Because CO_2 is a waste product of cell metabolism, it is continually being produced in the body and moved into the bloodstream. To prevent a toxic condition of the blood called **acidosis,** when there is an increase in CO_2 levels, we breathe more rapidly to carry the excess gas out of the body in expired air, as in panting during exercise. In contrast, when we breathe in too much oxygen, perhaps due to hyperventilation during an anxiety attack, we may "pass out." While unconscious, the negative feedback mechanisms will take over, causing us to breathe more slowly and deeply, conserving some of the carbon dioxide to balance out the increased O_2 levels and prevent **alkalosis** (a great way to help someone who is hyperventilating is to get him or her to breathe into a paper bag, thus conserving some of the CO_2 to balance the excess O_2 breathed in).

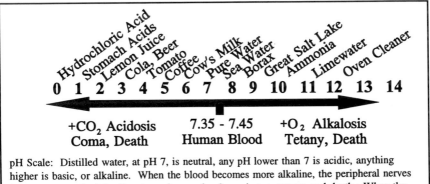

pH Scale: Distilled water, at pH 7, is neutral, any pH lower than 7 is acidic, anything higher is basic, or alkaline. When the blood becomes more alkaline, the peripheral nerves become overexcited, leading toward muscular & respiratory tetany, and death. When the blood becomes too acidic, the central nervous system is depressed, leading to coma, and death.

Regulation of Body Temperature

Since humans are warm-blooded creatures, we can regulate our body temperature rather than relying on the external environment to control it. Maintaining a constant body temperature as well as a specific volume and chemical composition of body fluids is very important to the normal functioning of our bodies. Chemical reactions and enzyme functions require a certain temperature range to be effective, and too high or low a temperature will kill off our cells. Thus we have many negative feedback mechanisms to help control body temperature. If we become overheated, the blood vessels in our skin relax and open up, or **vasodilate**, bringing warm blood to the body surface to be cooled. We can also perspire through our sweat glands, allowing the moisture on the skin surface to evaporate, cooling us further. If the body temperature is lowered too much, those skin capillaries **vasoconstrict,** or become narrower, to limit blood flow to the skin and keep the heat in our bodies. Cold also causes us to "shiver," an uncoordinated contraction of our skeletal muscles that generates heat as a byproduct of muscle metabolism.

Important, also, is an understanding of the effect of thermal treatments on other systems of the body, including the circulatory, respiratory, nervous, endocrine, and muscular systems, as well as metabolism and immunity. We will discuss these effects in more detail in the sections dealing with the application of heat or cold to the body.

Hyperthermia and Hypothermia

As a note of caution as we marvel at the efficiency of the body's protective mechanisms, let's have a few words about thermal injuries to the human body - times when the body can't cope with extremes of temperature. In some instances, the body's rate of heat production becomes greater than its ability to dissipate excess heat. This condition of elevated body temperature is referred to as **hyperthermia.** Often due to inadequate fluid and/or electrolyte replacement during exercise in hot weather, we can experience **heat cramps,** characterized by fatigue, excessive sweating, and muscle cramps. Treatment can include massage, PNF stretching and ice massage to relieve the cramping, as well as rehydration by ingestion of lots of cool water, salads, fruits, and/or electrolyte replacement beverages. A little more dangerous is the condition known as **heat exhaustion,** also often caused by inadequate fluid replacement, which is characterized by symptoms such as headache, nausea, hair erection on the upper arms and chest, chills, unsteadiness and fatigue. Often the skin is pale and cool, with profuse sweating, and the pupils may be dilated, with the pulse rapid but weak. Caution is advised in this case, which might result in shock symptoms, and sometimes a doctor's care is necessary to monitor kidney function and provide fluid replacement. Immediate care of shock symptoms of shivering and weak pulse includes covering the person with a blanket, and elevating the legs to encourage the blood flow to return to the heart. At the level of **heat stroke** we find a complete failure of the body's heat control system, with dehydration being an important factor. Symptoms such as incoherent speech, acute confusion and aggression, followed rapidly by unconsciousness, and an absence of sweating signal that this is an **emergency!** Get the person to a hospital quickly -

intravenous fluids are required to restore fluids and electrolytes, and the body's critical functions must be monitored.

In other conditions, however, we find that the body's rate of heat loss is greater than its ability to generate heat, resulting in lowered body temperature. This is known as **hypothermia.** This is common in inexperienced athletes who run the second half of a long race much slower than the first half, or inexperienced mountain climbers caught in winter storms without adequate protection. Causes include inadequate clothing, exposure to cool or cold environmental temperatures, low rate of heat production, or sweating combined with fatigue. Symptoms can include shivering, euphoria, disorientation, or intoxication. Treatment by wrapping the person in blankets will tend to bring the core temperature back up to normal. If the shivering is replaced by lethargy, muscle weakness and antagonistic behavior, this is an **emergency,** and the person should be referred to a doctor or hospital immediately to check on vital functions! In a condition of either hyperthermia or hypothermia, if there is any question about the mental alertness of the individual, it is important to monitor them through periodic questioning (asking for name, age, location, date, etc). It is unlikely, but possible, that a client would experience one of these conditions during a hydrotherapy treatment, so take note. Prevention is always best, but be aware of contraindications to treatments or poor reactions to them. Be prepared to take steps to help the client recover a normal homeostatic balance, including, but not limited to, ending the treatment, encouraging rest and the drinking of fluids, and making sure the person is warm, dry, and comfortable.

Classes of Physiological Effects of Water Treatments

Thermal physiological effects, obtained when we apply water at temperatures above or below normal body temperature, can be very powerful in healing. It is interesting to note, though, that a **difference in temperature** will have more of an effect on the body than the actual temperature of the environment. To illustrate this idea, try the following experiment. First place one hand in a warm water bath, while the other is in a bath of cold water. After the hands have become accustomed to these temperatures, place both hands in a bath at a temperature midway between the two. You'll probably notice that this water feels warm to one hand and cold to the other! We can also obtain effects on the body from **mechanical** stimulation (water striking the body surface) as in whirlpools, douches, sprays, and frictions. Thermal and mechanical treatments can be combined to intensify the effect on the body, as in a warm whirlpool bath or a cold mitten friction. And because water is the universal solvent, it is important in **chemical** interactions when used as an irrigation of a body cavity, as in a colonic irrigation, enema or vaginal douche, or swallowed as a nutrient. Because the thermal effects are so important in hydrotherapy (remember that **moist** heat or cold has a more powerful effect than dry, due to water's superior conductivity), let's look at what happens when we apply heat or cold to the body surface.

Primary Effects of Local Heat Application

The local application of heat to a specific body area will have several predictable primary, or direct effects on the body. First we'll notice **diaphoresis** - perspiration in the area will be increased to combat overheating. Along with this loss of water, there will be a loss of certain salts and nitrogenous wastes through the skin. Heat has a tendency to **speed up metabolism**, since the rate of all chemical reactions is increased in the presence of heat. According to van Hoff's Law, the velocity of simple chemical reactions increases two to three times for each rise of 10°C. Increased metabolism in muscles will tend to **decrease muscle tonus**. We find that pain due to muscular tension (which has been estimated at 70-90% of all pain felt in the body) will be relieved, so heat application will have an **analgesic** effect.

The smooth muscle tissue in the blood vessels of the skin will also relax, resulting, as we mentioned before, in **vasodilation** and **hyperemia** (reddening of the skin due to high concentrations of blood). Because heat application stimulates blood flow to the area, the **heat does not penetrate very deeply** (no more than 1.0 cm) into the tissues, but is confined to the skin and subcutaneous areas because the warmed blood is carried away

---

Effects of Local Heat Application
↑ Tissue metabolism
↑ Temperature of local skin area
↑ Diaphoresis and loss of salts
↑ Blood flow to area - derivation
↑ Temperature of body
↑ Migration of leukocytes
Vasodilation and hyperemia
Shallow penetration of heat
↓ Muscle tonus, ↑ Dexterity
Analgesic, sedative effect

---

by the increased blood flow. Thus the whole body can be warmed as a result of a hot foot bath. Because of the nature of the shifting of fluid concentrations in the body known as the **hydrostatic effect**, drawing blood toward the skin in one area of the body by local vasodilation will tend to drain fluid and congestion out of deeper tissues, resulting in the phenomenon of **derivation.** Remember that we're dealing with the body's defense mechanisms. When you sprain an ankle or cut a finger, you'll see these same results - **hyperemia, heat, and swelling**. Another defense mechanism, perhaps not as easy to note, that happens along with this increased blood flow, is an **increased migration of white blood cells**, or leukocytosis, into the tissues, to clean up metabolic waste products and debris from damaged tissues.

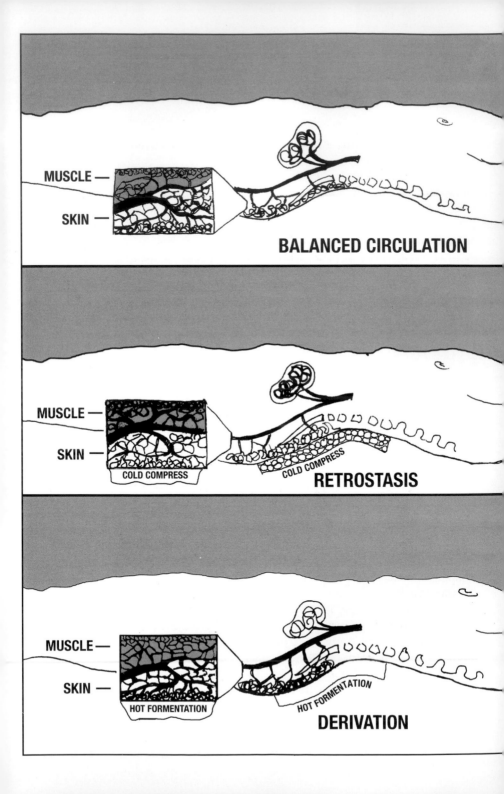

Primary Effects of Local Cold Application

The direct, or primary effects on the body of a local application of cold will be almost the opposite. The muscles will have an **increased tonus**, while at the same time there will be a **decreased dexterity.** If you've ever tried to fit a key in a car door lock in snowy weather, you'll understand this idea -you could probably drive the key completely through the door, but it's almost impossible to fit it precisely into the keyhole! And rather than vasodilation, we note that cold application produces **vasoconstriction,** resulting in **ischemia and blanching,** or pale skin due to diminished blood flow to the area, and a **decreased leukocytosis.** **Cold has a much deeper penetration** into the tissues as there is no influx of fresh warm blood to combat the cold influence. Because vasoconstriction literally drives blood out of the area, into deeper or more distant tissues, we see the phenomenon called **retrostasis** in action. This primary action of cold application is a reversal of the effect of derivation found in local heat applications, and results in fluids and congestion being forced out of constricted peripheral skin capillaries and into the deeper tissues of the internal organs. This obviously relates to a protective mechanism that conserves body heat by preventing its loss through the skin.

Effects of Local Cold Application
↓ Tissue metabolism
↓ Temperature of local skin area
↓ Diaphoresis and loss of salts
↓ Blood flow to area - retrostasis
↓ Local inflammation and swelling
↓ Body temperature
↓ Migration of leukocytes
Vasoconstriction and ischemia
Deeper penetration of cold
↑ Muscle tonus, ↓ Dexterity
Lessens spasticity in multiple
   sclerosis and Parkinson's disease
Anesthetic, numbing effect

We also find a **decreased rate of metabolism** in the tissues where cold is applied, which oddly enough also results in pain relief, but through an **anesthetic** effect: it numbs the nerve endings. This can be very useful in acute injury situations accompanied by pain, where an application of heat would cause a worsening of the symptoms. Remembering the acronym **RICE** (standing for "**rest** the injured area, apply **ice,** wrap with a **compression** bandage and **elevate** the injured limb above heart level") is helpful in situations of traumatic injury, especially within the first 24-72 hours. The RICE application not only prevents excessive bleeding and swelling and numbs the pain, but the ice limits metabolism and waste product build-up in the tissues, which can cause secondary hypoxic injury. This increases the rate and efficiency of healing.

Limiting swelling has an added benefit: studies have shown that the amount of scar tissue laid down in injured tissue is directly related to the amount of swelling present. While scar tissue formation is vital to repair of torn tissue, excessive scar tissue can limit range of motion in a healed joint, leaving it prone to re-tearing, causing future injuries. Scars can also shrink over time, causing pain and stress in the surrounding normal tissues.

Cold water application is very beneficial in the immediate treatment of burns, where it numbs the pain (keep applying it until the pain doesn't return when the cold application ends), decreases secondary tissue damage, and hastens healing. Note that in cases of both acute injury and burns, **immediate ice application** is best: the sooner it is applied, the more pronounced the beneficial effects. An important thing to remember though is that, due to the decreased circulation, there is a **danger of frostbite** (tissue death) from an extended application. A good rule of thumb is to **limit ice applications to no more than 15-20 minutes without a break,** but repeat the ice application often.

Contrast Applications

A **contrast** application of alternating heat and cold can be more comfortable than cold by itself, and is a very powerful treatment, utilizing the primary effects of both temperatures. Alternating derivation and retrostasis gives us the best effects of both heat and cold application, increasing the local blood flow by up to 100%. Heat application will bring fresh, oxygenated blood to the area to begin healing and carry out toxic waste products and debris. It is followed by the cold influence which will limit pain and swelling, while it slows the metabolism which causes the buildup of waste products. Swift healing and pain relief are the most obvious results of this powerful contrast effect known as the **circulatory whip**, or **vascular flush**. The relative lengths of application can vary, but an effective recipe is 3 minutes of hot water immersion, followed by 30 seconds to 1 minute of cold application. Begin with heat and end with cold, repeating the sequence 6-8 times, allowing approximately ½ hour for the whole treatment. Application can be by means of alternating water baths of hot and cold, applying a heating pad followed by ice massage, following a hot shower with a cool rinse, or many other treatment combinations.

Reflex, or Consensual Effects

Studies have shown that the effects of heat applied to the skin at most penetrate no more deeply than 1.0 cm, being carried away by the increased blood flow, and the effects of cold, even though penetrating more deeply, are driving increased circulation into the internal organs. How can we then affect those internal organs, beyond the simple circulatory effects of retrostasis and derivation, when we make a superficial application of heat or cold? A closer look at the effect of thermal applications to the skin leads us to the autonomic nervous system, and the concept of **reflex effects.** Although the skin surface has many millions of nerve endings, the viscera, or internal organs, contain relatively few (a section of skin the size of a quarter contains some 144" of nerves and 1,300 nerve cells in addition to 36" of blood vessels, 100 sweat glands, and over 3 million cells - the internal organs contain many fewer nerve cells and no sweat glands). Through the central nervous system we find a link, known as a **reflex arc**, where effects on the viscera are passed through neural pathways to be felt in the skin overlying that organ. For example, when someone has appendicitis, there isn't much sensation in the appendix, which has few pain-sensing nerve endings, but pain is often felt in the skin and reflected in muscle tension of the lower right abdomen, which lies directly over the appendix. These reflexes can work in reverse as well - when we apply cold to the skin overlying the appendix, we can reduce heat or swelling and relieve pain from that inflamed organ. While the reflex relationship is often between an organ and the skin overlying it, there are some additions or exceptions, such as the skin of the hands and feet, as well as the head, being in reflex relationship to the brain.

Reflex, or consensual effects, may be classified in three categories. They may be defined as **vasomotor**, having circulatory system effects - how the hot or cold stimulus affects the smooth muscle tissue of the blood vessels. They also may be categorized by hot or cold effects on the smooth muscle tissue of

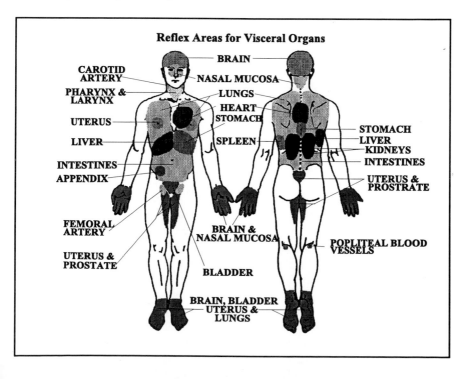

Reflex Areas for Visceral Organs

the viscera, referred to as **visceromotor,** or muscular. And they can also have an effect on glands, and thus on **glandular secretions**. For example, prolonged heat applied to the skin overlying the abdomen has been shown to result in decreased intestinal blood flow (a vasomotor effect), decreased intestinal motility and lessened tonus in the stomach (visceromotor - muscles relax with heat application), and decreased acid secretion in the stomach (relaxed stomach and intestines do not stimulate digestive glandular secretions.)   A prolonged application of cold to the same area will have the opposite effect - increased intestinal blood flow and motility (very effective in the case of constipation) and increased acid secretion in the stomach. Short alternating applications of heat and cold to the skin have a stimulating effect on the organs in their reflex areas, making contrast a very powerful healing procedure.

Reflex Effects in Hydrotherapy

Prolonged heat to the:

1. One extremity causes vasodilation in contralateral (opposite side) extremity
2. Abdominal wall causes decreased intestinal motility and blood flow, decreases acid secretion in stomach, inhibits digestion & stomach or intestinal cramping
3. Pelvis relaxes muscles of pelvic organs, dilates blood vessels constricted by cramping, increases menstrual flow
4. Chest (especially the center & left side - over heart) increases heart rate, decreases force of contraction and blood pressure
5. Chest relaxes bronchial muscles, relieves congestion through derivation
6. Trunk relaxes ureters or bile ducts to relieve renal or gallbladder colic
7. Kidneys in back and lower abdomen in front increases urine production (increases metabolism and filtration in kidneys, and relaxes urinary bladder)

Prolonged cold to the:

1. Trunk of an artery produces contraction of that artery and its branches
2. Skin over nose, back of neck and hands causes contraction of blood vessels of nasal mucosa - good for nosebleed, or **epistaxis**
3. Chest area over the heart slows heart rate and increases stroke volume
4. Skin of abdomen causes increased acid secretion in stomach and intestinal motility and thus increased intestinal blood flow to absorb digested nutrients
5. Pelvis stimulates contraction of pelvic muscles, including normalizing uterine **subinvolution** (restores uterus to normal shape & size after childbirth)
6. Thyroid gland contracts its blood vessels and decreases its function
7. Hands and scalp contracts blood vessels in brain (migraine remedy)
8. Inflamed joints, bursae and acute traumatic injuries causes vasoconstriction, decreased inflammation and relief of pain, and speeds recovery

Brief cold to:

1. Chest, with friction or percussion, first increase respiratory rate, then induce deeper, slower respiration
2. A reflex area of an organ, (see preceding diagram) accompanied by percussion, will increase functional activity of that organ
3. Precordium (skin over heart) causes increase in heart rate and stroke volume
4. Hands, face and head causes increase in mental alertness and activity
5. Skin (as brief as 30 seconds) in a warm environment causes a general peripheral vasoconstriction

General Effects of Heat Application

Now that we've explored the physiological effects of local applications of heat to particular body areas, we must look at what happens when heat is applied generally, by means of full immersion baths, multiple fomentations or vapor baths to the full body. When the whole body is affected, it must respond, not simply to elevated temperatures in specific tissues, but to a rise in the body's core temperature. Many of these effects will be similar to local applications, but note that there will be a few differences. In the attempt to cool the body, peripheral blood vessels in the skin will dilate to increase heat loss through radiation, conduction, and evaporation. As a result, there will be an increase in the rate of blood flow, perhaps as much as 400%! The pulse rate will increase 6-10 beats per minute per degree Fahrenheit rise in temperature, and the stroke volume will decrease: if we think about the heart beating at a faster rate, it doesn't have time to fill up as fully as normal, so the amount of blood being pumped with each beat will be less. We find an initial rise in systolic blood pressure (which measures the force with which the blood pushes against the artery walls when the ventricles

---

Effects of General Heat Application

- Muscle tension decrease
- Stroke volume decrease
- Initial rise in systolic blood pressure, then fall
- Lowered diastolic pressure
- Peripheral vasodilation
- Pulse rate increase
- Increased respiratory rate-hyperventilation
- Alkalosis can lead to tetany, chest oppression, panic
- Increase leukocytosis
- Increase blood volume, dilute
- Increase perspiration leads to dehydration, thick blood
- Salts loss through skin, aids in kidney disease

---

contract), followed by a drop back to normal or lower. We also find a lowered diastolic blood pressure (measuring the resistance of the vessels to the force of blood when the ventricles are relaxed). The difference of these two numbers is the pulse pressure, which is increased by general heat application. Pulse pressure is also increased by arteriosclerosis, where the systolic pressure rises more than diastolic, and in aortic valve insufficiency, where the diastolic pressure falls while the systolic pressure rises.

An increase in the respiratory rate is another result of a general application of moist heat, rising 5-6 respirations per degree Fahrenheit rise in temperature, in an effort to cool the body. **Hyperventilation** can result, creating an imbalance between oxygen and carbon dioxide in the blood, and this overbalance of oxygen (alkalosis, or an increase in blood pH) can lead to tetany or spasm of the muscles, oppression in the chest, and excitement. An effective remedy for alkalosis and tetany is to hold the breath, or breathe into a paper bag to allow carbon dioxide to accumulate to balance the blood pH.

Not only does the pH of the blood change, but the numbers of certain cells are increased. The leukocytes, or white blood cells, increase in number and move from the bloodstream into the tissues in the case of an artificial fever. This increase actually peaks several hours after the conclusion of the fever, and is similar to what happens during a natural fever - a mobilization of the body's defense systems. There is also a shift of fluids from the tissues into the blood, which initially increases the blood volume and dilutes it.

Increased perspiration is another result of the body's efforts to cool itself. This water loss results in a lowering of the fluid volume, with the blood concentrated and "thick," and also results in a loss of salts, urea, uric acid, creatinine, phosphates, sulphates, and lactic acid through the skin. During conditions of kidney impairment, excretion of waste products through the skin can be beneficial in preventing a toxic condition of the bloodstream, so full body hydrotherapy treatments can be very useful in patients with nephritis if **fluid intake is maintained** to prevent concentration of toxins in the blood.

General Effects of Cold Application

The intrinsic, or primary effects of prolonged cold application are basically depressive, including lowered core temperature, metabolism, heart rate, respiration, and sensation, slower circulation and digestion, and increased muscle tonus accompanied by a slow reaction time and decreased dexterity. An interesting illustration of these effects is the so-called **diving reflex** in children: you've probably seen newspaper reports of children who've fallen into icy water for an extended period of time, and seem to have simply shut down their systems and stopped breathing - when they're returned to the air, everything seems to start up again! When the body is overheated, as in a fever situation, cold application

---

Effects of General Cold Application

- Decrease core temperature
- Decrease metabolism
- Decrease pulse, respiratory rate
- Decrease sensation, anesthetic
- Slow circulation & digestion
- Increase muscle tonus
- Slow reaction time, dexterity
- "Tonic" to overheated body
- Slow cancer growth
- Use in cryosurgery, cryostretch cryokinetics
- Stimulate function of extensor muscles in spasticity, aids vision, joints, mood

will bring the body back into homeostatic balance, as a **tonic** treatment. Hypothermia has also been used in treatment of severe pain and to retard the growth of cancer, as well as in cryosurgery, cryostretch, and cryokinetics. **Cryosurgery**, where ice is used to lower core temperature, circulation, and metabolism, has been used in open heart surgery and surgical amputation of diseased limbs. **Cryostretch**, where ice is applied before stretching muscles back to their normal resting length after injury, and **cryokinetics**, where injured joints are exercised after prolonged ice application slows metabolism and limits swelling to guard against secondary hypoxic injury, are being used more and more to rehabilitate musculoskeletal injuries.

Moist cold application, both locally and generally, appears to have a beneficial effect in the case of spasticity of upper motor neuron lesions, including multiple sclerosis, stroke, Parkinson's disease, and post-operative spasticity. The cold seems to stimulate function in the extensor muscles of the body which are being inhibited by spasm in the flexor groups. Studies have also shown improvement in impaired vision, joint dysfunction, impaired sensation, and depressed mood in patients with these lesions.

Reaction

Often when we use thermal hydrotherapy techniques, our aim is to stimulate the negative feedback mechanisms, causing the body to react to a stimulus. Understanding this phenomenon of **reaction** is very important in successful water therapy treatments. When the body is subjected to a certain amount of stress, it responds with an alarm reaction. This stimulates strengthening of the body by gradually increasing the speed and efficiency of its negative feedback reactions, making the body able to successfully withstand more frequent and stronger stresses. As the heat-regulating negative feedback mechanisms of the body react to a cold stimulus to maintain thermal and circulatory homeostasis, we find the reaction passing through **three phases: circulatory, thermic and nervous.** When we splash our face with cold water, the initial circulatory vasoconstriction is followed almost immediately by vasodilation, accompanied by hyperemia in the skin. Other circulatory effects include slowing of the heart rate and a slight increase in blood pressure. In the thermic phase, metabolism is increased to heat the area in reaction to the cold application. And through stimulation of the nervous system, we note an increased tone in the muscles, along with a feeling of calm wakefulness and well-being.

If we apply too much stress at any given time, however, those homeostatic defense mechanisms will be overwhelmed, causing injury to the body. This leads us to the concept of **contraindications,** times or conditions in which it is either inadvisable to use certain treatments, or those treatments must be modified. Babies and children, older, ill, fatigued or convalescing patients, or those with drugs or alcohol in their system will not be able to respond as effectively as normal healthy people, and this must be taken into consideration.

Reaction to a cold stimulus can help to strengthen our vital forces. We must be careful, however, to watch for signs of an **incomplete reaction**, including gooseflesh, chilliness or shivering, cold hands and feet, or cyanosis (blue color) of lips, fingers and skin. These effects may or may not be accompanied by nausea, or a feeling of "fullness" and pressure in the head. In a case of incomplete reaction, the therapist must end the treatment, and use some method to warm up the client, such as a hot foot bath or wrapping them in blankets. Often cold, or **tonic** treatments are preceded by warming treatments, since most people respond more favorably to cold following heat applications or exercise. We can also use a mechanical stimulation, such as friction or percussion, along with the cold treatment. Interestingly enough, the use of **friction with cold not only increases the effectiveness of the tonic treatment, but for people sensitive to cold, it is much more pleasant.** We know that when people move from a warmer climate to a colder one, over a period of time we consider that their "blood has thickened," or they have adapted to their new environment. We use this natural adaptation mechanism to modify a person's sensitivity to cold, strengthening the body by using modified cold treatments repeatedly over a period of time. Finishing off hot showers with gradually cooler rinses, or a series of rubdowns with a cold loofah mitt or salt paste will allow the body to acclimatize to tonic treatments. The Polar Bear Club, whose members swim distances in icy water, have taken this adaptation to an extreme.

Contraindications to Heat Application:
Burns, bleeding, acute inflammation
PVD (peripheral vascular disease)
Diabetes, Raynaud's or Buerger's disease
Cancer
Cardiac disorders, hypertension
Person already overheated or dehydrated
Psychological problems
Inability to communicate, impaired sensation
Babies, elderly, drugged, unconscious people

Contraindications to Cold Application:
Cold hypersensitivity, fear of cold
Impaired peripheral circulation (PVD)
Diabetes, Raynaud's or Buerger's disease
Cardiac disorders, hypertension
Person already chilled or debilitated
Psychological problems
Inability to communicate, impaired sensation
Babies, elderly, drugged, unconscious people

Reaction to a hot stimulus, while it can be very beneficial, can also have an unhealthy effect on the body. More often the unfavorable effect will be a result of a full body application of heat, such as a wrap or steam bath rather than a hot fomentation applied to only one area of the body (although it is possible to burn the skin with an application that is too hot). The person receiving treatment may find muscles becoming too relaxed, to the point of fatigue and lethargy, or conversely there may be muscle twitching. There may be a feeling of dizziness, faintness, disorientation, rapid pulse or nausea, due to drastically lowered blood pressure. These effects can be combated by application of cold compresses to the head, or perhaps to the heart (to stabilize pulse rate), but if these measures do not solve the problem, the person must be taken out of the treatment. Dehydration and compromised kidney function are common results of heat treatments, which can easily be prevented by making sure the client **drinks plenty of water** to replenish the losses from sweating. Also note for the person that it is **inadvisable to eat a large meal** immediately before the treatment, since heat application to the abdominal area inhibits digestive processes, causing the food to remain too long in the system, and will also diminish the effectiveness of the treatment. Making sure the person **voids the bowels and bladder** before treatment will ensure greater comfort, and offset the effect of increased fluid consumption. Taking the **vital signs** (pulse, temperature, and blood pressure) before and during the treatment can help the therapist monitor for a negative reaction. Lastly, remember that any treatment utilizes the body's energy resources, which must be replenished - counsel the person to **rest** after the treatment to recuperate.

Keeping all of this basic information in mind, we'll discuss some common hydrotherapy treatments in the following chapters. Included in each will be **effects** (what normally happens in the body during the treatment), **indications** (situations where this treatment would be beneficial), **contraindications** (when not to use the treatment or when to modify it), and cautions or **special considerations.** Some of the treatments you can easily do for yourself. Others require a "therapist" to prepare the materials and assist the person into and out of the treatment. It's also nice, and sometimes necessary, to have an outside person to monitor vital signs, note and rectify a poor reaction to the treatment, and generally just "be there" for whatever might be needed. Welcome to the wonderful world of natural healing with water!

LOCAL HEAT, COLD AND CONTRAST TREATMENTS

General Notes for Treatments

Please read this before attempting any of the following techniques, and frequently refer back to the general contraindications, indications, effects, and special considerations for hot and cold treatments outlined in Chapter 1.

The intensity, duration and frequency of treatment depends on the effect you want - remember that children or weak, older or sick people are more sensitive to extremes of temperature, and may need a more moderate temperature or shorter treatment - keep checking to avoid burning or chilling. Diabetics, paralyzed or unconscious people, or those with respiratory, heart or circulatory problems or edema are especially at risk. Bony areas are more sensitive to temperature extremes than more fleshy areas. If the person (a baby, or an anesthetized or unconscious person) cannot indicate discomfort, be cautious with extremes of temperature and check the skin often.

Do not apply heat where there is danger of hemorrhage (bleeding) or cancer, and avoid spreading infections, or aggravating burns, bruises, or broken skin. Do not leave ice on the skin longer than 15-20 minutes, and check the skin during a cryotherapy treatment (it should be red rather than white) to make sure you are not encouraging frostbite. The person should be warm and comfortable during an ice treatment (the ice treatment area is very localized).

Explain the procedure and what effects the person might expect. Have all your equipment ready so you can stay with the person, both for his or her comfort and so that you can check for a poor reaction. Avoid getting clothes wet, so that the person can be dry and comfortable when the treatment is ended. Encourage fluid consumption and rest before resuming activities.

Fomentation

This is your basic moist heat treatment, easily applied, using towels or other cloth (wool tends to hold heat more effectively than other fibers when wet, but is often scratchy, cotton is more comfortable) soaked in hot water. It is very effective for relaxing muscle tension and giving pain relief locally, relieving internal congestion via derivation, and encouraging healing. **You'll need** a pot with hot water (and a means of keeping it hot), insulated rubber gloves, fomentation towels, dry towels, and some ice water in a basin. Following is a list of the steps you'll take in applying fomentations.

1.   Use a dry towel to protect the skin if the fomentation is too hot.
2.   Wring a towel out in hot water, using rubber gloves to prevent burning your hands.

3.   Apply the folded towel to the treatment area. A towel folded into several layers will hold heat much longer than 1 thickness.

4.   Cover with dry towels to insulate and apply a cold compress to the head to prevent overheating, if necessary.

5.   Change the fomentation every 3 - 5 minutes, checking to see that the skin is not being burned.

6.   Total duration of treatment: 20 minutes.

7.   End with a cold towel, briefly applied (perhaps briskly rubbed over the area), to restore homeostasis. This step is not vital if you'll be following the fomentation with massage or some other treatment.

Paraffin Bath

This is not literally a hydrotherapy treatment, but it is a commonly used method of applying heat to specific body areas. The paraffin wax is mixed with oil to prevent it from sticking to the skin or hair. It is often used to relax, warm and soften hands or feet preparatory to manicures, pedicures, or massage. It is also used therapeutically for arthritis in joints, or in cases of bursitis, fibrositis, tenosynovitis, or joint sprain after the acute phase is past to aid in restoration of normal joint function.   It takes an hour or more to melt the paraffin before use -don't allow it to get too hot! You can buy prepared paraffin and heating tubs for this purpose. Do not reuse paraffin, as it will become very dirty (or you can clean perspiration from used paraffin by placing it in boiling water for a few minutes, then cooling it down until the paraffin has rehardened. To sterilize the tank, heat it to a temperature of 180 - 200° F). **You'll need** heated paraffin wax that has been blended with a small amount of oil (preferably in a paraffin bath or slow-cooker on low to maintain the temperature), and plastic wrap and cloths to cover after dipping to retain the heat (and perhaps some safety pins to hold it together). You can also dip a hand or foot a few times into the bath to develop an insulating layer, and then keep it submerged for a brief time period.

1.   Remove jewelry, clothes, etc from the area to be treated.

2.   Wash and dry the treatment area thoroughly.

3.   Dip the body part or "brush" wax over the area 6 -12 times, cooling slightly in between. As you dip a hand in and then let it cool before re-dipping, you'll find a protective "glove" developing, which helps to insulate the skin. If you choose to brush the wax on, you must work quickly, as the wax will harden on the brush.

4.   Wrap with plastic wrap and cover with a towel to insulate.

5.   Duration of treatment: 10-20 minutes. Temperature range 122-130° F. Paraffin does not conduct heat as well as water, but you still can get burned, and heated metal jewelry can burn as well. Some skin areas, such as the front of the wrist, are more sensitive to heat - take the paraffin off that area and have ice handy in case you burn yourself.

6.   Remove the paraffin. Cool down the area with a dip in cool water.
7.   The paraffin, after removal, can be squeezed to develop hand strength.

Castor Oil Pack

We have Edgar Cayce (the "sleeping prophet") to thank for our information on this treatment. The castor oil pack is not literally hydrotherapy, but is a very effective **long-term mild heat** treatment, acting as a **stimulant** to the immune system and metabolism and as a **vulnerary**, encouraging healing from an external application. Castor oil comes from the castor bean of the palma christi plant - you might be familiar with its laxative effects when taken internally. When applied externally as a pack, it is an effective treatment for atonic constipation, peptic ulcer, or colitis (apply over abdomen), prostate or female pelvic problems (apply to low abdomen, groin, sacrum and inner thighs), or arthritis (apply over the affected joint). Cayce also suggests its use in cases of very localized cancer and non-acute appendicitis, but be very cautious in these cases, and never apply heat to an inflamed or swollen appendix (the heat won't feel good - apply ice instead, and see a doctor immediately). **You will need** 4 ounces of castor oil, flannel to absorb the oil, a sheet of plastic to protect your clothes or bedding, a source of mild heat, an old towel to insulate, and some baking soda mixed with water to clean up with afterward. You might also want some safety pins to hold everything together.

1.   Spread out your sheet of plastic and lay 2 or more layers of cotton or wool flannel on top.
2.   Soak the flannel in 4 oz warm castor oil.
3.   Flip the flannel & plastic over, so that the **oil-soaked flannel lies directly on the skin** over the abdomen or other area (the skin over the afflicted organ), and is covered with plastic.
4.   Cover with towel and heating pad on low heat, or another mild heat source. Be sure the heat is not too intense: since the treatment is long, it's important not to overstimulate the body.
5.   Duration of treatment: 1 - 8 hours.
6.   Skin should be cleansed afterward with water and baking soda (1 tablespoon : 1 quart) to prevent skin rash.
7.   The pack should never be washed, but can be reused for up to a year if stored in freezer, reheated before each use.
8.   You can try the packs in a series of 3-4 consecutive nights, then rest for 3-4 nights, then repeat. Another school of thought suggests using the packs daily as long as the problem persists. To make a series of packs more effective, try ingesting 2 teaspoons of olive oil nightly.

Hydrocollator/Silica Gel, Chemical, or Kenny Pack

This method of applying moist heat to a specific area requires an investment. These canvas packs filled with silica gel come in different sizes and shapes, and retain the heat much longer than a fomentation, so they don't require changing during the 20 minute treatment. You can also buy a hydrocollator tank that heats the water to 160°F and keeps the packs moist. Note that silica gel packs that dry out become brittle, and are very difficult to re-use - they should be stored in water (or wrapped in plastic and placed in the freezer if they won't be used for awhile). It takes an hour or so for the packs and water to heat up when you turn the tank on. **You'll need** heated silica gel packs, towels for insulation and drying, and a cold compress.

1.   Use a **minimum** of 3 - 4 thicknesses of dry towels between the skin and the pack to insulate, **so the skin won't burn**.
2.   Lift pack from tank with tongs and place on towels over area to be treated. Or you can use fitted terry cloth covers.
3.   Cover pack with dry towels to insulate from air.
4.   Total duration of treatment: 20 - 30 minutes.
5.   End with cold procedure to restore homeostasis.

Hot Foot Bath

This treatment is wonderful for general body heating and relaxation, as well as preventing or healing the common cold or flu. It increases the blood flow through the feet, helping to relieve the tiredness and achiness from standing for long periods. The derivation effects can draw congestion out of the head to relieve headache or nosebleed, and out of the chest and abdominal and pelvic regions to relieve congestion there (add a teaspoon of powdered mustard, ginger, or cayenne pepper to the water to increase this effect). *You could also make this a hot arm bath! **You'll need** a pot or basin that the feet will fit into comfortably, hot water and a thermometer, ice water and a cloth for a cold compress, and a towel to dry the feet. You may want a blanket to wrap the whole body in to induce sweating and false fever for a cold or flu treatment.

1.   Wash feet, submerge in a pan of hot water for 10 - 30 mins. Dish basins or small washtubs work well.
2.   Temperature range 100 - 115° F. (Can start at low end of range and gradually add hotter water).
3.   Apply a cold compress to forehead, back of neck.
4.   Finish with cold water rinse, dry the feet thoroughly.

Ice Pack, Cold Compress, Ice Cup Massage, Slush Bucket

These local cold treatments are great for sprains, strains, bruises, dislocations, and other overuse or traumatic injuries exhibiting the cardinal signs of inflammation: redness, heat, swelling, pain, or loss of function. They are also great for acute arthritis, tendinitis, or bursitis, hemorrhage, or a burn. Use as part of RICE application (rest, ice, compression, elevation) in acute injuries. (See Appendix B). Women experiencing painful menstrual cramps can use the ice cup to massage the area of the 2nd lumbar vertebra on the right side for pain relief. **You'll need:** for the **compress**, wring out a cloth in ice water. For the **ice pack**, fill a plastic bag with crushed ice (this is nice because it molds itself around injured joints). For **ice cup massage**, fill waxed paper cups 2/3 full with water and keep them in the freezer, ready for use - stick a popsicle stick in the center when they're half frozen for a non-icy handle - peel away the cup edge to massage the affected area with the ice. For a **slush bucket**, fill a small tub with icy water enough to cover the affected part (often a hand, ankle, foot) - be sure the ice doesn't all melt away or the water will not be cold enough.

1. Use a fomentation prior to application if the person is sensitive to cold and condition is not acute.
2. For ice massage, move the ice cup directly over the skin. Or, for variety, soak the body part in a slush bucket.
3. For an ice pack, apply a dry cloth, then a plastic bag filled with crushed ice, a frozen gel pack, or an icy compress. (An interesting variation - a bag of frozen peas or corn molds well around injured joints). You might want to cover it with a towel to insulate.
4. Duration time: **not more than 15-20 minutes at a time**. Care must be taken that the person does not get frostbite or nerve damage in the treated area. If you are giving a cold compress (cloth wrung out in cold water), you must frequently dip the cloth back into the ice water and reapply it to maintain the cold application.
5. Re-apply cold treatment often during the first 24-72 hours after injury. Rule of thumb - 20 minutes on, followed by 20 minutes off, & repeat.

Moist Abdominal Bandage / Heating Compress

This heat treatment begins with application of a **cold** compress, which is insulated to prevent heat evaporation. As the body reacts to the cold stimulus, the compress is gradually heated up via natural metabolism, to provide a long-term, mild, moist heat treatment. The only **heat source is the person's own body heat.** It is great for tense muscles (apply to specific area), sore throat, laryngitis, or tonsillitis (apply to throat with or without camphor, menthol or other aromatic oil), rheumatism, chronic arthritis or synovitis (apply to joints with or without medication), chronic bronchitis, whooping cough or pneumonia (apply with or without medication to chest). The moist abdominal bandage, applied to the abdominal area, is useful in insomnia, central nervous exhaustion, constipation, "morning sickness" of pregnancy (don't allow the woman to become overheated, however), or other gastro-intestinal disturbance. **You'll need** a cloth and some ice water for the compress, another cold compress for the forehead, and a large towel (and perhaps a plastic bag) to insulate. You might also want safety pins to hold things in place, and a hot foot bath to warm the person prior to beginning.

1.   The person should be warm - you can start with hot foot bath, etc
2.   Apply the compress - a wet towel (single thickness) wrung out in **cold** water - to the abdomen or other area of the body.
3.   Add dry towels to insulate and secure them by pinning.
4.   Duration time: 1-8 hours. Treatment must be complete to be effective - i.e. the cold compress must be warmed through or dried by body heat.
5.   Check for signs of an incomplete reaction (blue lips and fingertips, shivering, headache, goose bumps, etc) and take steps to insure the person will end up warm, dry and comfortable.

Whirlpool Bath / Jacuzzi / Hot Tub (Varying temperatures)

This is a bath to a specific body area, often the limbs and joints of the extremities. Some whirlpools are large enough for full-body immersion, but therapeutic baths are generally smaller. This treatment combines water of the desired temperature mixed with an air stream to provide thermal and mechanical stimulus to the area treated. **Heat** is relaxing, stimulating blood flow for healing non-acute injuries (sprains or fractures after the first 48 hours, post-operative rehabilitation, amputation stumps, muscles strains, arthritis). **Cold** tones muscles, reduces inflammation and metabolism (peripheral nerve injuries, burns: use a saline solution to cleanse dead tissue to prevent infection at burn site).

You'll need a whirlpool tub, step stool, and a towel to dry off with. Treatment time is 10-30 minutes, perhaps briefer with a cold whirlpool. See Contrast Treatment for a recipe for alternating hot and cold - you'll need 2 tubs.

Jacuzzis and hot tubs are often in the warm to hot temperature ranges (see page 10). There are generally several jets around the pool, which diminishes the force of an individual jet, so they usually aren't as powerful as a therapeutic whirlpool, although they can be very relaxing. They are often large enough for the full body (or several), exhibiting effects similar to treatments found in the next chapter, so review the contraindications listed in Chapter 1- effects of general heat treatments. A common problem with hot tubs is that they are unknowingly set at too high a temperature, or people remain in them too long, resulting in dizziness, fainting, or becoming dangerously weakened. Those with heart or circulatory problems are also at risk. Remember that treatments in the hotter temperature ranges should last no more than 10-20 minutes or so, and you should have cool water nearby for a compress or for sipping.

Sitz Bath (Varying Temperatures)

This bath to the pelvic area leaves the legs, arms, chest and head outside (sometimes given in a specially-constructed sitz bath tub).   You can also use a large metal washtub that is large enough to sit in, or you can do this treatment in a regular bathtub.   This treatment specifically targets the pelvic organs (prostate, uterus, bladder, colon) and the effects will be related to temperature and duration.   Generally **heat** will stimulate pelvic circulation, relax muscles and relieve pain (low backache, menstrual cramps, chronic bladder infection, prostatitis, intestinal cramping, chronic pelvic inflammatory disease). **Cold** will slow metabolism, increase muscle tone, and stop bleeding (cancer, hemorrhage, hemorrhoids, atonic constipation, returning uterus to normal after giving birth). **You'll need** a sitz tub, rubber mats to avoid slipping on wet floor, hot foot bath, cold compress, a source of hot water and ice, and a towel.

1.   Have the person take a hot foot bath before and/or during treatment.
2.   Assist the person into the tub. To safely control the descent, grasp the person's wrists and lean away with your back straight, bending at the knees to avoid injury, as you lower them into the tub. Water should cover the entire pelvic region.
3.   Apply a cold compress to the forehead if using a hot sitz, or place the feet in a hot foot bath with a cold sitz.
4.   Assist the person out of the tub, have them shower and dry thoroughly.
5.   If it's a hot sitz, end with cooling procedure; if it's a cold sitz, make sure the person is warm to begin with, and does not get chilled.
6.   If it's a contrast sitz, try 3 minutes in hot, 1 minute in cold (you can use a loofah friction mitt to rub the pelvis during the cold phase). Repeat 3 times, beginning hot, ending cold. Pat dry.
7.   Duration of treatment: 2 - 12 minutes.

Alternating Hot/Cold (Contrast Treatments - Circulatory Whip)

As the name implies, this treatment alternates a hot application with a cold one. You can combine fomentations with compresses, hot foot baths with ice water baths, hydrocollator with ice cup massage, or any other ideas you might have. General guidelines are to begin with heat and end with cold, repeating several times.   Generally the heat influence lasts longer than the cold (maybe 3:1). You'll get the most beneficial effects of each treatment, with the negative effects minimized - the circulatory whip is an extremely effective healing agent!

1.   Begin with **heat**: 3 minutes.
2.   Contrast with **cold**: 30 seconds to 1 minute.
3.   Repeat 8 to 12 times for optimum results.
4.   Begin with heat, end with cold.
5.   Pat dry and warm the person.

6.   Try small plastic tubs for hand or foot contrast, ice cup massage with
          fomentations or hydrocollator, contrast sitz baths, whirlpools, or ?

Fluxion to the Spine

   Here is a type of contrast treatment, specifically aimed at the spine and the
paraspinal muscles. This is a crossroads area for the nervous system - all of the
peripheral nerves enter or leave the spinal cord here between the base of the
occiput and the sacrum, and it is an area that holds a lot of muscular stress as
well. "Fluxion" refers to a quickening of the rate at which blood passes through
a body area. Fluxion to the spine provides a cleansing "circulatory whip" effect,
carrying out toxic byproducts of metabolism through the veins and lymphatic
system, while arterial blood flow is increased, bringing in oxygen and other
nutrients to this all-important spinal area. It's wonderful for paraspinal muscle
tension, back pain, emotional stress, and head congestion, leaving the person
feeling calm, clear-minded, and energized. **You'll need** a source of hot water,
insulated rubber gloves, a folded towel that just covers the spine from the base
of the head to the sacrum, a dry towel to cover, a cold compress for the head,
and an ice cube or ice cup.
1.   The person lies face down, with **cold** to the head, **fomentation** for feet.
2.   Wring another fomentation out in hot water using rubber gloves. Fold
          up the towel to retain heat and focus on the spine only.
3.   Place this fomentation along the spine from the occipital ridge to the
          sacrum for 3-4 minutes. If the fomentation is too hot, a dry towel may
          be spread underneath to protect the skin.
4.   Remove fomentation, rub an ice cube up and down spine 5-10 times.
5.   Steps 3 and 4 are repeated 6 - 8 times, ending with ice.
6.   Dry the person thoroughly. Treatment lasts about 30 minutes.

Vapor Inhalation, Facial or Foot Steam

   Water vapor inhalation is wonderful for bronchitis, sinusitis, colds, or
respiratory flu, while the steam on the face also relaxes muscles and opens pores
to cleanse the skin. You can enhance the effectiveness of the steam by the
addition of herbs or essential oils to the boiling water, such as eucalyptus,
peppermint, menthol, wintergreen, or pine needle oils or witch hazel to help
soothe the mucous membranes of the respiratory passageways. The heat also
relaxes the smooth muscles of the bronchioles. Eucalyptus, chamomile, basil,
spearmint and peppermint can be added to facial vapors for all skin types. Oily
skin would beg astringents like lavender, lemon grass, orange peel, rosebuds, or
rosemary, while emollients for dry skin include clover, rose, and primrose.
You'll need a facial steam unit, pot of boiling water or a teakettle (to which
you've added the herbs if you want them), an umbrella for over your head, and

a towel large enough to completely cover umbrella, head, & steam source, to hold in the steam. Breathe in the steam for 20-30 minutes, finishing with a cool compress or a splash of cool water to the face. Take care that the steam does not scald you, as steam burns can be very nasty (remember latent heat of vaporization!).

Water vapor applied to the **feet** is a great way to alleviate the problem of sweaty, smelly feet. Lay a wooden rack over the steaming pot and rest your feet on it for 20 minutes. They'll perspire quite a bit, but after a brief cold soak and a brisk towel rub, you'll find that they tend to sweat less and smell much sweeter. You might need to repeat this treatment several times in extreme cases.

FULL BODY HEAT AND TONIC TREATMENTS

General Information

Make sure you are familiar with the effects and contraindications relating to Local and General Applications of Heat or Cold from Chapter 1. Also review cautions listed before Local Heat, Cold, and Contrast Treatments at the beginning of Chapter 2. Make sure you are aware of any medical problems or medications the person is taking, and be prepared to take steps to keep the person healthy and comfortable. Full-body treatments have the potential for more powerful healing effects than local treatments, but be aware that the negative side effects can also be more powerful!

Russian Bath / Steam Cabinet

This is a full body steam bath with the person's head outside of the cabinet. This requires a specially-constructed cabinet with a source of steam, a chair or bed to lie upon, and an opening to allow the head outside. You can construct your own using PVC pipes, clamps and a tarp (ask at a hardware store), or you can buy individual "mini steam baths" that come with their own steam source. Remember to look for contraindications before beginning this treatment (check in Chapter 1 - General Applications of Heat). Leaving the head outside allows the person to breathe much more easily, since extremely moist air interferes with gas exchange in the lungs, so in this way the Russian bath is superior to a fully-enclosed steam bath or sauna. It also allows the pulse and temperature to be monitored, and compresses to be applied to the forehead or neck. You can, however, give a medicated Russian bath in which the head is enclosed, adding medications to the steam (see Vapor Baths in Chapter 2) for relieving inflammations in the nasal passageways. Maximum temperature 120°F (maximum 200°F for sauna = dry heat). **You'll need** tea or water to drink beforehand, a steam cabinet, a towel to sit or lie upon, a cold compress for the head, a thermometer, a watch (for pulse), and a towel to dry off with. People with minor heart problems might apply an ice bag over the heart to steady its beat.

1. Count the person's pulse, blood pressure (see Appendix C), and/or take the temperature. Suggest emptying bowel and bladder for comfort, and drinking fluids before the treatment to avoid dehydration.

2. Have the person lie on a towel (with a bolster under the knees if lying on the back) in the steam cabinet, with the head outside, and wrap the neck with a small towel to seal in the steam.

3. Apply cold compress to the forehead (ice bag to heart if pulse is above

80 beats per minute). Give water to drink as needed, through a straw.
4.   Check the pulse & temperature every 5 minutes, and change the compress frequently.
5.   Watch for rapid pulse, dizziness, or fainting.
6.   Duration of treatment: 5 - 10 minutes.
7.   Cool (perhaps with cool scotch douche or shower to wash off impurities that have been flushed out) and completely dry the person after the procedure. Record the time, ending pulse and blood pressure, temperature and reaction. Counsel rest and fluid intake after treatment.

Hot Blanket Pack / Herbal Wrap

The hot blanket pack is actually a full-body version of the fomentation - a moist heat treatment, with multiple fomentations applied under and on top of a person lying supine. The person, covered with the fomentations, is then wrapped first in a rubber sheet, and then wool blankets to insulate. A cold compress is applied to the forehead, and changed frequently throughout this **20-30 minute** procedure. The fomentations may be soaked in an herbal tea, rather than plain water, to make this an herbal wrap (see chapter on Herbs in Hydrotherapy or an herbal book for herb suggestions). A version of the herbal wrap found more commonly in luxury spas makes use of thick layers of unbleached muslin sheets instead of towels for the fomentations. This wrap elevates the body temperature (false fever), increases blood volume by draining internal tissues and encouraging blood flow to the skin, induces perspiration with an accompanying loss of certain toxins through the pores of the skin, lowers blood pressure after an initial rise, and relaxes muscle tension. It is known for its **detoxifying** properties (especially the herbal wrap - certain herbs can increase this effect), and its loss of water weight, relaxation and stress relief effects.

    You'll need a **table or bed** with a **bolster or pillow** to put under the person's knees, **2 large wool blankets** (army blankets work well), **2 large rubber sheets** or pieces of plastic (enough to wrap completely around the body from the neck down and fold under the feet), **many old towels or large unbleached muslin sheets** for fomentations (enough for several thicknesses to wrap around the body), a **cold compress and a basin** filled with ice water to refresh the compress, a **bath towel** to wrap around the person's neck to prevent drafts, a **large pot filled with hot water** or herbal tea, **herbs in a large tea bag** to make the tea, **insulated rubber gloves** for wringing out fomentations, and a cup of **drinking water with a straw** in case the person gets thirsty during the wrap and **hot tea for drinking** before and after the treatment. You might also want some **soft music** to aid in relaxation.
1.   **Have the person drink** hot tea to begin warming. Suggest emptying bowels, bladder, and taking a cleansing shower prior to the treatment.

2. **Make the herbal tea** for the wrap (or just use hot water), and place the fomentations in to soak.

3. **Meanwhile,** set up the table or bed in this way: Place the bolster or pillow about where you think the person's knees will be. Now lay down the wool blankets with one blanket hanging off one side of the table and the other blanket off the other side. Decide which end will be for the person's head and lay down the neck towel ready to wrap around the neck. Make sure the blankets hang off the foot end of the table so that they can be folded under the feet later (they won't need to wrap around the head - this side can be even with the end of the table). Lay the rubber sheets down on top of the blankets in the same manner.

4. **When the person is undressed and ready** for the treatment, wring out the fomentations as dry as possible, and spread them quickly on the prepared table. The person should then quickly lie on top (the cloths cool down quickly, but make sure the person's skin is not burned!). Cover the person with fomentations or muslin sheets (sheets can be placed centered under the person then wrapped around - with arms <u>up</u> wrap from one side, then with arms <u>down</u> wrap from the other side, to cover the arms as well). You can add an extra fomentation around the feet or center of the body, if desired, to increase temperature.

5. **Wrap the rubber sheets and blankets** from the sides of the table snugly around the person, tucking in under the feet, and wrap the towel around the neck to prevent drafts. The effect is now rather like a mummy, with only the head exposed (you can also wrap a towel around the head to increase the insulation.)

6. **As you wrap**, try to avoid getting wrinkles in the material - lying on folds for 20 minutes is a bit uncomfortable. Also try not to wrap too loosely - there might be air pockets that can feel chilly.

7. **Place the compress** on the forehead, refreshing this several times in the ice water basin throughout the 20-30 minute wrap. For thirst, give some water (the straw makes sipping easier).

8. **Stay with the person** during the wrap, talking softly if desired - some people get a feeling of claustrophobia and this will give confidence and encourage relaxation (you can also allow the arms or feet to remain outside of the pack if there is a feeling of being too closed in). You can check the carotid (neck) pulse every so often to monitor. You may also want to gently massage the face or feet to aid relaxation.

9. **Complete the procedure** with a brief cold treatment. Cold mitten friction (page 41) is particularly effective. Dry the person completely, then advise resting for 20 minutes or so. Encourage fluid consumption to replace water lost through perspiration.

Wet Sheet Pack

This full-body treatment is interesting because it can be a **cooling, neutral or heating pack**, depending upon how long you allow it to continue. It is similar in application to the local application called the heating compress in that the wet sheet is actually a cold compress wrapped around the entire body, with evaporation regulated by wool blankets wrapped around it. The only source of heat is the body's own resources reacting to the cold stimulus. In the initial stage (usually not longer then 5-10 minutes - review incomplete reaction in Chapter 1) the body will feel the effects of the **cold** compress, useful in lowering fever, or in conditions of general weakness. In the second stage (perhaps lasting half an hour, depending on the speed of reaction), as the body begins to heat the compress, the temperature becomes more **neutral**, which is very calming to the nervous system in cases of insomnia, anxiety, delirium, or restlessness. In the third and last stage, since the moisture cannot evaporate into the air, the body temperature begins to rise, and the person becomes **overheated** and begins to perspire. At this stage, it is vital to change the compress to the forehead often so the brain doesn't become overheated. This stage can be helpful in recovering from colds or flu, breaking fevers, drug or tobacco detoxification, soothing bronchitis, colitis or arthritis, and can help relieve some strain on the kidneys in chronic nephritis by allowing some toxins to be released through the perspiration.

    You'll need a table or bed for the person to lie upon, a bolster or pillow for under the knees, a large sheet that will cover the body and cold water to wring it out in, a cold forehead compress and a basin of ice water for refreshing it, 2 large wool blankets, 2 large rubber sheets, a neck towel to prevent drafts, and drinking water with a straw, to relieve thirst during the treatment.

1.   **Follow** the steps outlined for body wraps under the Hot Blanket Pack (above), **except** instead of the hot fomentations beneath and around the person's body, you'll use the large sheet as a cold compress wrap. After wringing the sheet out in the cold water, spread it out on top of the blankets and rubber sheets. Have the person lie on top of the wet sheet, raising the arms. You'll fold one side of the sheet over the body, then have them lower the arms to fold up the other side, enclosing arms and body, and tuck the lower end over the feet. Wrap up the rubber sheets and blankets, again tucking in the feet, and wrap the neck towel snugly to avoid drafts. Again, avoid wrinkles or air pockets as you wrap, since they might be uncomfortable.

2.   **You might wait** until the person is feeling hot before you apply the forehead compress.

3.   **Encourage resting** and drinking of fluids after the treatment.

Salt Glow

This is a wonderful, invigorating treatment that exfoliates the dead skin cells from the body's surface, stimulates blood and lymphatic flow, stimulates the metabolism, and leaves one feeling refreshed and clean. I have found it a great way to finish off a full body peloid (clay or fango) treatment - the clay is a bit hard to clean off completely, so the salt glow finishes the job. Try the treatments at the beach, rinsing off in the ocean water. **You'll need** a box of sea salt granules (perhaps adding a bit of iodine) and a bit of water in a bowl to make a gritty paste, water to wash off the salt (or do it in the shower), and a towel to dry off with afterward. You might suggest the person **not shave** immediately beforehand, because the salt will sting!

1. **Pour** a container of salt into basin, **moistening** with water to make a paste. (Adding too much water will make salt water, not paste!) Paste can be slightly heated in microwave, or use **hot** water for comfort.
2. **Make sure** the person is **warm** to begin the treatment (it's good to do this treatment in a warm room).
3. **Wet** the person's skin, then begin circular rubbing with salt paste moving slowly centripetally (toward the heart), starting with extremities. **Give friction** to tolerance. You can rub with more force over foot, knee and elbow calluses to soften them.
4. **Avoid** open cuts to prevent stinging, but spend extra time on callused areas (heels, knees, elbows).
5. **Then** do the chest, back, and buttocks (the abdomen and face may be omitted if desired).
6. **Remove the salt thoroughly** by shower, spray, or hose. Be sure the **salt does not remain too long on the skin**, because it will irritate it.
7. **Dry off** thoroughly.

Cold Mitten Friction

Using cold water-soaked loofah or terrycloth mitts, this is an invigorating massage, useful for acclimatizing cold-sensitive people to tonic treatments, and building up the immune system's resistance. It stimulates circulation and metabolism, increases white blood cell activity and antibody production, and stimulates neuromuscular and vasomotor tone, as well as cleansing the pores of the skin. This is good for convalescence after illness or fever, stress, anemia, and hyperthyroidism. **You'll need** two loofah or terrycloth mitts, a basin of cold water, and a towel to dry off with.

1. The person should be warm to begin the treatment, in a warm room.
2. Wring the loofah mitts out in cold water, & rub vigorously over skin, starting with extremities, then chest and back, one area at a time.
4. Rub dry briskly with the towel, making sure the person is warm.

Dry Brushing

You can use loofahs, a natural bristle body brush with a handle, a sisal strap, or natural sponges for dry brushing techniques. Dry brushing will exfoliate dead surface skin cells and stimulate the blood and lymphatic circulation. It can be used for people are extremely sensitive to cold to adapt them to the cold mitten friction, and later to more intense tonic treatments. (Remember, tonic treatments are not meant to chill the body, but to stimulate a **reaction** of the immune system to strengthen it without overwhelming the body's defenses. This is why we make sure that the person is warm and comfortable to begin and end the treatments). Dry brushing the skin in a centripetal direction (toward the heart) stimulates the lymphatic system to cleanse toxins out of the tissues. Performed daily, it is a good accompaniment to colon-cleansing procedures and fasting. Be sure not to continue it indefinitely, however, since it is subject to adaptation, and will cease to be effective if you don't allow resting days.

Spray, or Needle Shower

Multiple needle spray or shower heads in this treatment allow water to strike the body from many different directions at once. You need a specially-equipped needle shower to experience this (check out spas in your area). This is a wonderful cleansing and relaxing treatment when given using warm to hot water, and an invigorating one when using colder temperatures. Using alternating hot and cold gives vascular exercise (vasodilation alternating with vasoconstriction) and relieves fatigue. Oddly enough, taking a **cold shower on a cold day will tend to conserve body heat** (retrostasis drives the blood internally to prevent heat loss through the skin), and a **hot shower on a hot day will tend to cool the body down** (derivation draws blood to the skin capillaries to radiate heat away from the body). Dr. Olav Blomquist originated an alternating hot and cold **allergy spray** (beginning with an increase from 100-110°F for 3 minutes, then rapidly decreasing to 85°F for 2 minutes, repeating 3 times with hotter hot and colder cold temperatures each repetition, followed by friction drying and a 20 minute rest period) for the treatment of rhinitis, hay fever, and asthma.

Percussion Douche (Scotch Douche or Blitzgus)

This treatment combines thermal and mechanical effects - water massage as a **column of water** strikes the body, combined with varying temperatures, depending upon the effect desired. A fairly heavy force of water pressure is effective, but it's wise to **fan** the water to somewhat diminish its force over more delicate areas of the anatomy, such as bony prominences, the abdomen, and the low back (kidney) area. Women will probably find it preferable to cover the breasts and genitals with an arm to avoid the water striking those areas altogether, while men should cover the genitals with the hands. The therapist should avoid douching the head and neck also. **Cold** water will have a tonic effect (good for finishing up heat treatments), while **hot** water will be more comfortable and relaxing, or you can try a **contrast** of hot and cold. The effect of the water striking the body surface will speed up blood and lymphatic flow to aid healing and stimulate metabolism. Avoid bruises, painful swellings, or areas of broken skin. **You'll need** a hose with a control nozzle, connected to a source of hot or cold water under pressure (a tub or shower - it's good to work in a reasonably large enclosed, tiled area, as this treatment is very wet - be careful you don't slip)! You'll also want a towel to dry off with.

1. A douche is a column of water directed against the body. Temperature will vary due to effect desired (see page 10).
2. Begin at the foot (with the person facing away from you), pass up one side of the back of the body and back down to the foot to douche the other side. Then have the person turn to face you and repeat for the front of the body (covering the breasts and genitals with the arms to protect them).
3. Keep a finger in contact with water from nozzle to monitor temperature and fan the water over more delicate areas.
4. The direct force of the jet can be used on upper & middle back, buttocks and thighs, but water should be fanned over more sensitive areas, such as low back, back of knees, front of elbow, abdomen, etc.
6. Duration approximately 5 - 6 minutes. Dry the person thoroughly after.

Hubbard Tank

This treatment requires a specially-constructed full-immersion tub, which has adjustable bars for support during underwater exercise, and one or more jets which mix an airstream with the water for hydromassage. Temperatures can range from **cool** (for multiple sclerosis or Parkinson's disease sufferers), to **neutral** (with saline or brine solution for cleansing away dead tissue in burn victims or those with bedsores or pressure sores - decubitus ulcers), to **warm or hot** (to produce a mild fever and relax muscles in sufferers of arthritis). Burn victims, arthritis sufferers, and others find the water exercise vital for maintaining range of motion in injured joints supported by the buoyancy of the water, and for preventing deformities from scar tissue shrinkage. For weak, paralyzed, or injured people, one can make use of stretchers and mechanical lifts or hoists to lower them into and help them out of the tank.

BATHS

Herbal Bath

Consult an herbal (book dealing with healing properties of herbs) or the next chapter (Herbs in Hydrotherapy), to choose an herbal bath. The easiest way to prepare the baths is to obtain a "hops" bag from a beer and wine supply store or health food store, fill it 1/3 full (for a 7" X 7" square bag) and run **very hot water** over it. Adjust the bath temperature once the herbal properties have leached out (you can use the herb-filled bag as a sponge while in the bath to increase the effects). You can also buy essential oils of various herbs, a few drops of which can be added to a normal bath. Generally this bath would be in the warm to hot temperature range (maximum 110°F), for relaxation.

As an antidepressant, try bergamot, chamomile, jasmine, lavender, orange or rose in the bath. For a sedative, or relaxing bath, perhaps marjoram, rose, lavender, frankincense, sandalwood or chamomile would be good choices. Herbs for a pain relieving bath might include bergamot, chamomile, lavender, rosemary, nettle, pine, cayenne, cloves, eucalyptus, or wintergreen. Camphor, bay, nutmeg, eucalyptus, geranium, lemon or rosemary would tend to give a stimulating bath.

Apple Cider Vinegar Bath

This will detoxify by a drawing action similar to the effects of clay treatments. (Soaking fruits and vegetables in apple cider vinegar water helps pull out pesticide residue). For **muscle soreness and aching joints**, combine this bath with self-massage. While soaking in a warm bath to which one or two cups of apple cider vinegar have been added, slowly massage the entire body, starting with the soles of the feet. Gently but firmly squeeze and relax each part of the foot, working your way slowly up the leg to the hip; do likewise with the other foot and leg. Continue up the torso, then do hands, arms and neck, always massaging towards the heart. For the face, lightly pat the skin in an upward direction, avoiding pulling facial skin downward. Finish up with a fingertip massage in circular motions over the scalp and head (this is also a great tonic treatment for dark hair after shampooing). Rinse with a bucket of cold water to which ¼ cup of apple cider vinegar has been added. The vinegar smell will evaporate, but you can rinse thoroughly in clear water to wash the residue away.

A variation on this theme is the **apple cider vinegar and salt massage** -wrap coarse salt crystals in muslin or gauze, saturate with vinegar, and massage sore muscles. You can also apply this as a poultice, binding it in place and leaving it on for four or five hours at a time.

Epsom Salts Bath

Epsom salts, or magnesium salts, added to a warm bath will draw out muscle soreness as it relaxes the muscles, and cause a cleansing perspiration following the treatment. Add 1-5 lbs salts to the bath water and soak for 10-30 minutes. This bath is great for athletes' or "weekend warriors' " muscle soreness after a particularly grueling workout.   Edgar Cayce also recommended it for rheumatism, sciatica, arthritis, injuries, and incoordination.   He did note, however, that people with high blood pressure or heart difficulties might encounter problems due to the stimulating effect and the increase in blood circulation and heart rate, especially at higher bath water temperatures.

Oatmeal Bath

This bath is soothing for irritated skin conditions, such as eczema or mild sunburn, as well as for the scalp. Add a pound or less of uncooked oatmeal, enclosed in a hops bag (see Herbal Bath) to the hot water as you begin to fill the tub. After a couple of minutes, adjust the temperature so that it is in the tepid to neutral range (90-97° F) and use the oatmeal-filled bag to sponge the skin as you relax in the bath. Rinse thoroughly, and gently pat dry.

Spinal Bath

This bath is a wonderful tonic for the nervous system, and thus to the whole body, being excellent for calming and relieving tension as well. The bather lies in the tub with one or two inches of cold water from neck to coccyx. Ice may be added to lower the temperature. The feet and legs should be up and out, or preferably in a bucket of warm water. The person may be covered with a big towel if chilled. Always make sure the bather does not get chilled! (A hot bath to begin is good insurance against colds.) The bath may be taken for 15 - 45 minutes, or until the bather awakens (often people fall into a very refreshing sleep). The Spinal Bath should be ended with the Head Bath (described below), since it sometimes can cause congestion in the head..

The Head Bath

Pour cold water over the head 10-20 times so as to cool the brain. Those trying the spinal bath for the first time may feel heat and congestion in the head after the treatment, and this head bath quickly brings the temperature to normal. It may also be done as a treatment by itself, as it is good for toning the scalp, stimulating healthy hair growth (try adding nettles, bay or lavender to the water), and stimulating the brain.

Cold Bath

From the treatments of Kneipp, Preissnitz, and as far back as the Spartans comes the idea for using cold baths to harden the immune system, renew energy and sexual vitality, improve circulation with resulting reduction in heart attack, stroke and cold hands and feet, and strengthen skin, hair and nails. It involves taking a cold bath (55-70°F) on a regular basis, followed by a brisk rubdown with a towel to dry off. Those who are particularly sensitive to cold, or are debilitated or weak, or just beginning the cold baths, should keep the water at the top of the range, and bathe for 5-10 minutes or less (see cold mitten friction, salt glow, dry brushing, and hot shower ending with cold for further ideas in adapting to cold). As the body becomes stronger, longer and colder baths will be better tolerated and more effective. You can begin a cold bath by patting cold water on the forehead and over the heart to prevent shock, then stepping in with the feet and moving around to become acclimatized to the cold. Then submerge the legs for a few minutes, then up to the waist, and finally full immersion up to the head, taking several minutes for adaptation at each stage before progressing to the next. Be sure that the person does not become chilled, and make sure they end the treatment warm and dry (a brisk rubdown with a towel is often nice, perhaps followed by light exercise for a minute or two to rewarm the body).

Neutral Bath / Flotation Tank

This bath derives its effect from being as close to body temperature as possible, in the range of 94-97°F, so that there is very little stimulus to the nervous system. It is very relaxing, and is especially good for those who are overstressed and for calming psychiatric patients or the anxiety-plagued, who sometimes react adversely to extremes of heat or cold. The bath can last for 30 minutes to several hours (although with a longer treatment, you'll find the skin can become temporarily very waterlogged and wrinkled). It can also be very good for those with certain kidney or heart problems (under careful medical supervision) through making the blood less viscous, increasing heart pumping effectiveness, and relieving fluid retention.

A variation on this bath is the flotation tank, based on the experiments of Dr. John Lilly, who studied the effects of long-term immersion in water using his "sensory-deprivation" tanks. In the tank, the person floats in a neutral temperature bath, buoyed up by the addition of Epsom salts. The bath is enclosed in a tank which prevents the entry of sound or light, so that all of the senses can rest. A novice in this treatment might feel a little claustrophobia at first (the therapist will show how easy it is to let yourself out of the tank, which sets fears at rest), but most people begin to relax rather quickly, and the 30 minute to an hour treatment is a great meditation. In some flotation tank situations, films may be shown, illustrating someone perfectly performing an athletic skill. Because the tank is so relaxing, the mind can escape all of the excessive stimuli it normally has to filter out, and can focus on absorbing all aspects of the illustration, and resulting in improved performance of that skill later on. (The movie version of this treatment, in which the man stayed too long in the tank and regressed back to mankind's primeval origins, was highly unrealistic!)

Thalassotherapy - Sea Water Bath

From the Greek term for "sea" comes the name for this treatment, either (ideally) spending time at a thalassotherapy spa on the ocean, inhaling mists & taking various kinds of baths in clean ocean waters, or by putting sea water salts into a bath at your home. Sea water contains salts which can add a beneficial effect to the water treatments (see "Spa Therapy").   There are many spas along the coast of the Dead Sea, for example, that specialize in psoriasis and other skin treatments, as well as treatments for many circulatory and respiratory diseases. The Dead Sea has particularly high levels of salts in its water which can enhance the water treatments. There are many products available which contain these salts, as well as various seaweeds and ocean sands or muds.

HERBS IN HYDROTHERAPY

Herbal Glossary

Alterative (gradually restores health)
Analgesic (pain reliever)
Antibiotic (kills bacteria internally)
Antipyretic (febrifuge - reduces fever)
Antiseptic (destroys superficial bacteria)
Aromatic (volatile fragrance
  - clears nasal passages)
Astringent (dehydrates, shrinks tissues)
Balsamic (soothes)
Carminative (dispels gas)
Cathartic (purgative - evacuates bowel)
Counterirritant (skin irritant
  - reduces deep inflammation)
Diaphoretic (promotes sweating)
Diuretic (promotes urine flow)
Emmenagogue (promotes menstruation)
Emollient (soothes skin)
Expectorant (evacuates phlegm)
Laxative (evacuates bowel)
Nervine (calms nerves, tension)
Rubefacient (increases local circulation)
Sedative (reduces nervous tension)
Soporific (induces sleep)
Stimulant (quickens body functions)
Styptic (stops external bleeding)
Tonic (invigorates, strengthens system)
Vulnerary (heals wounds)

The use of plants for healing purposes is one of the earliest forms of medicine. From 1550 BC, when the Egyptians noted down herbal prescriptions for many diseases in the Ebers Papyrus, we have a scientific record of natural medicine. Through Hippocrates' treatments in 5th century BC Greece, and later in the Materia Medica written by Dioscorides in the 1st century AD and the Roman physician Galen's writings in the 2nd century AD, we find developments and adaptations of the earlier treatments. The Chinese, Indians, and Native Americans also handed down healing information through word of mouth, or in such texts as the Pen Tsao Ching (3400 BC) and Pen Tsao Kang Mu (1590 AD) from China, and Indian Ayurvedic texts. The peasants, too, developed treatments using locally available herbs. We have no records of these, though, since reading and writing were the province of the elite classes, and unavailable to the common folk. Although many records list male physicians by name, many of these unsung folk, knowledgeable in healing methods, were un-named women - midwives, nurses, "wise women," mothers - treating family, friends neighbors.

There are many choices of herbs or combinations that can be used for varying effects in an herbal wrap or herbal bath, in a tea for drinking, or as a local healing application by plaster or poultice (definitions below). The following is a very basic overview of some of the more common herbs used in hydrotherapy. Investment in a good herbal guide (or several) will be the necessary next step for those wishing to expand their herb use.

Don't be misled, however, by simplistic generalizations stating that herb use, because it is "natural," has no negative side effects. We saw in our discussion of water and its effects upon the body that there are always cautions and contraindications to the use of any therapeutic device. We are all different, having varying strengths and weaknesses, and any time you apply anything to the body surface or internally, changes will occur, some of which we desire, and some of which we don't. Some herbs (such as foxglove, containing digitalis, which is used to stimulate the heart in congestive heart failure patients) can be used therapeutically, but can cause death if too large a quantity is used. In many cases it is hard to know exactly how much of the active ingredients will be found in a given sample of the herb, so controlling the amount received can be a problem. Another example of a potentially dangerous herb is licorice: many people enjoy the flavor, and it can be useful for coughs, but those with heart or blood pressure disorders should avoid its use. The box on the previous page will give an understanding of some basic terms relating to herb use that will come in handy later on. Note that something can have both sedative and stimulant effects, for example, because they are not opposing qualities by these definitions.

Many herbs are heat, moisture, and light sensitive and will lose their healing essences if not properly prepared and stored. Teas, tisanes, infusions, decoctions, tea-soaked fomentations, plasters and poultices should be freshly made, as they will not keep for more than a day. Tinctures, elixirs and spirits, made using alcohol as a preservative, will keep indefinitely, but should be stored in sterile amber glass containers. Salves, ointments and flower essence oils may be kept in small quantities indefinitely in sterile, widemouthed amber jars, but should be smelled from time to time, as oils can go rancid. Dried or powdered herbs should be stored in a cool place in dry, airtight dark glass containers. Washed containers may be sterilized by boiling them for twenty minutes, then allowing them to cool and air dry. Aluminum, iron, tin, or other metals will leach into the herbs, so it's best to use glass, ceramic, or enameled containers, wooden spoons, and paper towels when preparing herbs.

Herbal Definitions

Decoction: Herbal ingredients extracted from roots and bark by simmering for 20 minutes or more. When making mixed decoctions, start roots first, then add barks, seed, herbs, flowers, and lastly spices gradually as they take progressively less time to extract the active principles.

Flower-, Herb-, or Spice- Essence Oil, Vinegar, or Water: Place flower or herb in oil, vinegar, or water base, and put it out in the sun in a clean glass jar to protect it from the elements. It will take a few days for the essential oils to diffuse into the base. You can make great "sun tea!"

Infusion, Tisane: The extraction of active properties of a substance by steeping or soaking, usually in water. More effective with leaves, flowers and delicate herbs. Dried herbs are, as a general rule, twice as potent as fresh, which have a higher water content. A tisane is a single cup type of infusion which is steeped only briefly, for immediate use. This type requires more herb to make a strong enough concentrate.

Liniment: Herbal extracts that are rubbed into the skin for treating strained muscles and ligaments, relief of arthritis and some types of inflammation. The extraction is accomplished with vinegar, alcohol, or massage oil.

Plaster: This is like a poultice, but the herbal materials are either placed between two thin pieces of linen, or are combined in a thick base material and then applied to the skin. Often used for strong substances, such as mustard, cayenne pepper, or ginger, which might blister the skin.

Poultice: A warm, moistened (with water, herb tea, cider vinegar, etc) mass of powdered or macerated herbs (sometimes oatmeal or flour is added to make a thick paste) that is applied **directly to the skin** to relieve inflammation, blood poisoning, etc. and to promote proper cleansing & healing. Can also be made of other materials such as clay or charcoal, and applied at varying temperatures.

Salve or Ointment: A preparation that can be applied to the skin and remain in place, due to its thick consistency. It's usually made by extracting herbs in hot oil, adding other active ingredients, then adding beeswax so that it will be solid at room temperature.

Suppository, Bolus: A semi-solid substance for introduction into the rectum, vagina, or urethra, where it dissolves. It often serves as a vehicle for medication. A **bolus** is a suppository made by adding powdered herbs to cocoa butter until it forms a thick pie-dough consistency. Shaped like a bullet, it's placed in the refrigerator to harden, and later allowed to warm to room temperature before using. Inserted into body cavities to treat various cysts, tumors, infections, irritations, etc.

Tincture (50% alcohol), Elixir (25%), Essence (10-20%), Spirit (10%): Highly concentrated herbal extracts, usually made with potable alcohol, taken internally, or applied externally as a liniment. Elixirs, essences and spirits are progressively more diluted with water.

Common Herbs in Treatments

Herbal wraps often make use of herbs that are emollients, tonics, nervines, and diaphoretics, or have pleasing or stimulating fragrances. Examples might include rose petals, chamomile flowers, lavender, comfrey leaves, orange or lemon flowers or peel, jasmine, clove, or various mints. **Healing bath** herbs can vary greatly, depending upon the intent of the bath. **Tension relievers** include catnip, chamomile, jasmine, mullein, rose, vervain, or violet. Herbs that **stimulate**, such as citronella (also good in candles to keep mosquitos at bay), mint, pine needle oil, calendula, lavender, rosemary, sage, nettles, or fennel can make a bath a good "pick-me-up." For **foot baths**, try agrimony, alder bark, burdock, lavender, mustard, sage, or witch hazel. **Vapors** more often utilize decongestants, astringents, aromatics, or stimulants, like eucalyptus, peppermint, wintergreen or other mints, menthol, witch hazel, or pine needle oil.

Natural First Aid

Having certain herbs or other natural remedies close at hand can allow quick and effective treatment of common maladies, and many of these you'll find in your kitchen cupboard, masquerading as spices! Others you'll have to look for at the health food store or in an herb catalog, but they're worth the effort. The following list is but a hint at some of the many uses for these natural substances.

Bay leaves, ginger, mint, wintergreen, cardamom, caraway, cinnamon, allspice, anise, and fennel are good for upset stomachs or relieving intestinal gas. Try drinking mint (or basil, a member of the mint family) or bay leaf tea for a stomachache or "morning sickness" of pregnancy, dabbing a bit of oil of wintergreen beneath your nose when nausea starts, eating ginger cookies before a boat or car ride to prevent motion sickness, or chewing fennel or cardamom seeds after dinner - the pleasant flavors also freshen the breath. **Parsley** is another great breath freshener, and high in vitamins A and C, calcium, and iron, as well. Anise can also help those with coughs, bronchitis, or asthma. Cinnamon also seems to be effective against diarrhea, botulism, staph, and various fungi. Ginger also lowers blood cholesterol, thins the blood, and has anti-cancer properties. Spread some crushed bay leaves around kitchen cupboards to repel cockroaches.

Apple pulp contains high amounts of a soluble form of fiber called pectin, which has a variety of beneficial effects on the body. It adds bulk to the stool, which makes it beneficial in cases of both diarrhea or constipation, soothing the intestinal walls and promoting normal bowel contractions. "An apple a day keeps the doctor away" may not be simply an old wives' tale - the pectin has been shown to reduce blood cholesterol, aid in prevention of colon cancer, help to control blood sugar levels in diabetes, and even help eliminate toxic heavy metals such as lead and mercury.

Chamomile makes a great relaxing tea of an evening - save the tea bags, allow them to cool, and apply to the eyelids to soothe and brighten tired and reddened eyes. The tea can also be used as a rinse to accentuate blond highlights in the hair (as can lemon juice - rosemary or vinegar rinses are good for brunettes). Inhalation of the tea vapors can relieve nasal stuffiness. Thinly sliced **cucumber** applied to the closed eyelids, soothes the eyes and helps minimize dark circles. A **rose hips** poultice is good for puffiness below the eyes (and also for the common cold!). **Witch hazel** is also useful for eyes - to reduce swelling, puffiness, and dark circles under the eye. Since it is an astringent, it is good in general for toning the skin and as a treatment for hemorrhoids, bruises, or stings. **Oatmeal** is very soothing for skin irritations - cook the oatmeal and either apply as a paste or strain and use the oatmeal water to soothe rashes and other skin itches or inflammations. A hot poultice made of **thyme** leaves and flowers, applied to pimples or boils, will draw them to a head to help healing. Try a few drops of **rosemary or jojoba oil** massaged into the scalp and hair for beautiful tresses.

Garlic (the "stinking rose") and onions not only taste good in foods, but are credited with germ-killing properties and can help to lower high blood pressure by inhibiting blood clotting, to help prevent heart disease. Garlic, in particular, is effective against colds, some influenza viruses, athlete's foot fungus, staph and strep bacteria, germs causing cholera, typhus and dysentery, and intestinal worms. If you're not a fan of garlic's aroma, you can buy "odorless" garlic capsules at the health food store (or chew parsley afterward). **Basil, licorice root, or parsley** tea acts as a mild laxative in cases of constipation. Try **apple juice** to help dissolve gallstones or kidney stones, or **cranberry juice** for minor urinary tract infections.

Coffee is not only the morning wake-up call for many people, but has been credited with relieving attacks of bronchial spasms in asthma sufferers. Since it tends to constrict blood vessels, the caffeine in coffee (as well as tea and chocolate) can be used to relieve the pain of migraine headaches. Coffee enemas (given rectally) have been prescribed for asthma and cancer (beware, though, since one can easily overdose on caffeine by absorbing coffee through the colon's walls). Try applying coffee-grounds water on the legs to help heal varicose veins. **Feverfew** is also helpful for migraines, as well as high blood pressure, menstrual cramps, and digestive problems.

Cayenne pepper is, oddly enough considering its fiery flavor, useful as a soothing remedy for the digestive tract (black pepper is **not**, however). It is also useful as a stimulant, as a gargle for sore throat, or internally to heat the body to break a fever through sweating or warm the tissues of a frostbite victim. Used externally in a poultice or liniment for sore muscles or sprains, cayenne be used to increase blood flow to an area, thus increasing heat, and reducing inflammation and pain. Cayenne (including paprika, which is a very mild form of the pepper) is very high in vitamins C and A, iron, potassium, and niacin. **Mustard and ginger** plasters also help stimulate blood flow to relieve congestion, relax muscles and relieve pain.   **Salt** water also makes an effective gargle for sore throat pain, and drawing it up through the nostrils (one at a time) can relieve a runny nose for an extended period of time.

Echinacea, while not normally found in most peoples' kitchen cabinets, is worth a trip to the health food store to obtain. It is valuable as one of the best blood purifiers, and is an effective antibiotic, as well as a stimulant to the immune system.   Swallow the capsules to abort a cold or the flu, help heal hemorrhoids, and detoxify beestings or snakebite.

Activated charcoal (you can buy it in capsules) is also great for bad breath, acid stomach or intestinal gas, or as an antidote to poison, due to its wonderful adsorption properties. You can use it, too, as a plaster for infected wounds or swellings, eyeball scratches (place over the closed eyelid - pain and inflammation relief is almost immediate, and vision quickly returns to normal), or in a bolus mixed with cocoa butter for ear pain. You can also heat the ear with a hair dryer on low, or a hot pad to speed up the pain relief in the ear.

Myrrh is very useful in gum irritation - just rub it over the affected area and gum pain or itching disappears!   **Clove oil** is a good antidote for a toothache, again applied directly over the painful area. Because of its germicidal properties, clove oil is also an effective ingredient in mouthwashes for sore throats. **Baking soda and hydrogen peroxide** are wonderful for preventing or healing gum disease by preventing bacterial growth and plaque buildup, when used as a toothpaste.

Arnica and **comfrey** (which contains the active ingredient allantoin) are good to have on hand to heal bruises and sore muscles fast. Apply mixed in a cream or oil base, as a poultice or tincture, available in health food stores or latin farmacias. Cold compresses soaked in **witch hazel, marigold or wintergreen** tea are effective in healing sprains (or try applying **parsley** leaves). Growing **aloe vera** in the garden or as a houseplant ensures that you have a ready remedy for sunburn or other burns, scrapes, or wounds. Cut off a tip of one of the fleshy leaves to release the mucilaginous juice, and apply it directly to the burn site. Keep reapplying as it dries to keep the area moist, relieve pain, and help it heal.

Australian tea tree oil is a natural antibiotic and fungicide. Mix a few drops with glycerin and apply it directly onto the itchy tissues to treat vaginal yeast infections - the relief is almost instantaneous. Called a "first aid kit in a bottle," it can also be used for athlete's foot, earache, wounds or burns, herpes lesions, or as an insect repellant. Unprocessed **honey** is also a fungicide and its antibacterial properties make it an effective ointment to apply to cuts and scrapes.   **Eucalyptus** has antibacterial properties useful for healing minor wounds, combating the flu virus or preventing bacterial bronchitis. Along with **horehound** and **slippery elm**, it is a common ingredient in throat lozenges, and is also used in chest rubs for loosening phlegm, and promoting free breathing.

POOL AND SPA THERAPY

Pool Therapy Physical Principles

In addition to its superior heat conducting ability, water has other properties which we can make use of in underwater, or pool therapy. First of all, it has weight, which we describe in terms of specific gravity, with pure water itself being the basis of comparison, or a **specific gravity of "1."** Anything less than "1" will float, while anything greater will sink in water to a certain extent, depending on the specific gravity of that material. Any impurities, such as various salts and minerals dissolved in the water, will increase its weight, thus affecting the following properties as well.

Water exerts **hydrostatic pressure** on the body surface, which is increased by greater depth or density. We can compare this idea with atmospheric pressure, exerted at fifteen pounds per square inch at sea level. Atmospheric pressure decreases with increased elevation above sea level, which we associate with a feeling of "lightness," and if we go below sea level, we get the opposite feeling, of "weightedness." As soon as we enter a pool of water, we feel it pressing in against our skin equally in all directions, and certain physiological changes happen in the body as a result. There is compression of the veins and lymphatic vessels, which increases venous and lymphatic flow. Hydrostatic pressure applies an inward force on the abdominal and thoracic cavities, which also increases the flow of blood back toward the heart, and in turn increases the stroke volume of the heart, perhaps as much as 24%.

Archimedes' Principle comes into play when we talk about the **buoyancy** of water: an immersed body is buoyed or lifted up by a force equal to the weight of the liquid displaced. Buoyancy modifies the effect of gravity by supporting some of the body weight, allowing earlier rehabilitation of musculoskeletal injuries or post-surgical conditions in which pain and secondary injury limit movement. It is also effective for rheumatoid- and osteo- arthritis patients, allowing them to do pain-free exercises, which help heal joint inflammation, give them more strength, and allow more freedom of movement. Since bone and muscle have a higher specific gravity than water, they will tend to sink more, but are offset by the air volume in the chest and the body's fat stores, which, because of their lower specific gravity, will aid the buoyant effect. Pool exercise can also take advantage of the **viscosity**, or cohesive force of water, which gives slight resistance to underwater movement in any direction. This is the most significant force against movement parallel to the surface. Associated with viscosity is **hydrodynamic force,** or the **resistance** to movement through water. Water resistance increases disproportionately with the speed of movement and the shape and size of the moving object: a small, slow-moving streamlined object will encounter less resistance than a large, blunt object moving more quickly.

Values and Indications

Pool Therapy Indications:
(Temperatures will vary)

- Early traumatic injury rehab
- Early surgical rehabilitation
- Improve morale
- Save time & money
- Avoid "pain / spasm" cycle
- Relieve stress & pain
- Aerobic, muscle fitness
- Arthritis, sprain, strain
- Fracture, tendinitis, bursitis
- Lordosis, kyphosis, scoliosis
- Paraplegia, polio, palsy
- Scleroderma, MS
- Congenital nerve defects
- Prosthetic stump prep
- Psychiatric conditions

Contraindications:
(Remember thermal cautions)

- Fever, systemic, skin infection
- Eye, ear, nose, throat infection
- Acute inflammation ("itis")
- Heart disease, arteriosclerosis
- High or low blood pressure
- Active polio or pulmonary TB

Pool therapy offers an opportunity to rehabilitate surgical patients, or those who have suffered traumatic injury, sooner and more effectively than with conventional therapy. In this way, it can improve morale, and save time and money (insurance companies should love this benefit!) with a speedier recovery. After surgery for tendon injuries, joint repair or replacement procedures, muscle damage, or bone fractures, exercise helps the damaged tissues heal much faster and more efficiently. Waiting six weeks or more for a broken bone to heal leads to muscle atrophy throughout the body, joint stiffness, and weaker bones, which would then require far more rehabilitation time. Likewise, common sports injuries such as knee or ankle ligament sprain, tendinitis, back spasm, or muscle strains, don't have to limit an athlete's training. Since athletes' morale suffers probably more than that of a non-athlete (many of us can often use a rest break!), many methods and tools have been developed to allow normal training exercises to be carried out in the pool. Buoyancy belts support runners in an erect position so they can "run" in the water, and webbed gloves and fins give water resistance to replace that of gravity in arm and leg exercises. You can even use plastic milk cartons, which when empty will float, to press under the water to give resistance for arm or leg exercises.

Warm water also has a sedative effect, aiding relaxation for tense and neurotic patients, and helps to avoid the pain - spasm - pain cycle by relaxing cramped muscles that would impede circulation. Arthritis sufferers, people with scoliosis or polio, scleroderma and fibrositis victims, those with peripheral nerve damage or neurological defects, and even paraplegics can benefit from the relaxation and buoyant support of the water while they move stiffened joints, stimulate circulation, and strengthen painful and often atrophied muscles. There is even some experimental therapy work being done with nerve-damage patients to restore a degree of nerve function by mimicking the walking cycle in the water, including the sensation of the heels striking the bottom of the pool, and the knee, ankle and hip movements involved.

Contraindications

As in all the treatments we have discussed, however, there are some conditions in which pool therapy is contraindicated, or where modifications as to temperature or length of treatment should be made. People with fevers, or a systemic illness such as the flu or a bad cold should either limit the length of time they are in the pool, or stay out altogether and wait until they have regained their health. Even healthy persons should note whether they feel undue fatigue or loss of appetite after sessions in the pool, and modify or discontinue pool activities for awhile. Those with acute inflammation of the joints, active joint disease, or neuritis might find that even pool therapy is too painful.

Since immersion in a pool increases peripheral blood flow and kidney circulation (why is it that we often feel that we have to urinate as soon as we get into a pool?), those with nephritis or other kidney disease would find this type of therapy too much of a strain on those organs. For similar reasons, pool exercise could be dangerous for cardiac patients, or people with very high or very low blood pressure. Eye, ear, nose, or throat infections, or active pulmonary tuberculosis are some other contraindicated conditions for pool therapy. Incontinent patients, with weak bowel or bladder control, should do their work in an individual Hubbard tank rather than in a communal pool.

Specifics for Pool Therapy

Many tools have been devised for assisting in pool therapy. For safety and support, pools may have railings, bars, or ladders to help people climb safely into and out of the pool, and to hold on to while performing exercises. For paralyzed or weak individuals, there may also be devices with slings to lower them into the pool, although these will be more commonly found in Hubbard tanks (see Chapter 3), for individual work. Non-skid mats are also very useful to avoid slipping in puddles around the pool area. To allow for underwater exercise, you can purchase (or make) weighted chairs, stools, belts or boots to resist the buoyant effect of the water. Foam belts can help keep a runner erect in the water for rehabilitation exercises that mimic running, but without gravity's stress on injured joints. Fins, floats, paddles, balls, and empty plastic bottles can give added resistance to underwater movements to strengthen specific muscles, and snorkels and masks will allow swimmers to maintain a balanced spinal alignment as they won't have to turn their heads continually to breathe when working face down.

Temperature ranges can vary, depending upon the activity. A warmer range of 98-100°F is effective in cases of spastic paralysis to relax muscles in spasm, and 92-95°F is good for isolated exercises. The water should be cooler (80-90°F) for active swimming, since there can be **no sweat evaporation** under the water to dissipate the heat generated from the aerobic exercise. Swimming in a pool that is too warm can lead to heat exhaustion or undue fatigue.

The treatment time can vary from 5-30 minutes or more, again depending on the activity, as well as the condition of the person being treated. A healthy athlete can train for an hour or more, whereas a debilitated paraplegic might not be able to do more than a few minutes of exercise. For anxious or restless people, 1-2½ hours relaxing on floats in a neutral temperature pool can relieve their stress.

Spa Therapy

"Spas" were originally named after the town of Spa in Liège, Belgium where mineral springs were first discovered in 1326. The term carried the meaning of a health resort possessing a **source of mineral waters**, where one can soak in, drink, or inhale vapors from those waters. While they are especially popular in Europe (Germany has over 200), where they are run by medical personnel and supported by government subsidies, unfortunately spa therapy is now often looked upon as quackery in the USA. We still have many resorts left over from their heyday before the advent of allopathic drugs, but the quality control is much lower than in Europe. You'll find some spas remaining (not all still operating) in Hot Springs Arkansas, Saratoga Springs and Clifton Springs New York, Marlin Texas, White Sulphur Springs West Virginia, French Lick Springs Indiana, Hot Springs Virginia, Fordyce Bath House Arkansas (now a park and museum), and many in California, Oregon, and Colorado. America has many so-called spas now, but the term is loosely used for many **luxury resorts**, which offer massage, beauty treatments, weight loss and diet modification, and back-to-nature retreats, but in most cases have no source of mineral springs.

Spa Classifications

Traditional spas can be classified as either thermal, saline, gaseous, or iron-bearing. In **thermal** spas, the water can be hot enough to burn the skin, and are often located near rivers, where cooler water can mix in with the spa water. You'll many times find several different pools of differing temperatures, depending upon the proportions of spa water and river water. Resorts are often built directly over the river and the source of the mineral springs, with some of the water piped into individual baths. **Saline** baths contain chlorides, sulfates and carbonates of sodium, potassium, calcium, or magnesium, and are often whitish or colored (such as the chlorides), or have obvious odors (such as the "rotten egg" scent of sulphur springs). **Gaseous** waters contain natural gases under pressure, such as carbon dioxide, hydrogen sulfide, radon (which is radioactive, but reputedly with healing properties), and are often bubbly. And waters that contain at least 10 mg iron per liter, which gives a reddish tint, are considered **iron-bearing** waters.

Effects and Indications for Spa Therapy

If one is submerged in a bath of mineral water, many of the effects will be similar to those of pool therapy described above, and the general effects of heat application (for thermal spas) from the first chapter. Remember that minerals dissolved in the water will increase the weight of the water, so you'll find **increased buoyancy, viscosity, and hydrodynamic forces**, as well as **increased hydrostatic pressure** upon the body surface. This will stimulate lymph and venous flow, allow one to float with ease, and give added resistance to underwater exercise. In addition, many spas offer **vapor inhalation** therapy to soothe the respiratory tract, and mineral ions may pass from water applied to the skin to **"transmineralize"** the body. Rheumatoid and osteo- arthritis and gout, anxiety and insomnia, tension headaches and fatigue, sinusitis, bronchitis and asthma (aided by inhaling vapors), gastrointestinal problems (helped by drinking sulfates and phosphates of magnesium and sodium for their laxative effects), eczema and psoriasis, and iron-deficiency anemia are all indications for spa therapy.

Peloids or Clay Therapy

Many spas also include treatments with peloids (mud or clay baths), which can be of three different varieties. Mineral mud, or **fango**, contains volcanic ash, mineral **sea muds** are made of finely-ground shells of sea animals, and organic muds or **peat** are made up of decomposed vegetable matter. Clay has a silicon base, containing also oxygen and aluminum, and often iron, magnesium, and many other trace elements as well, similar in makeup to the semiconductors used in computer technology. These modern ceramic materials, as well as clay, have been found to have a crystalline structure and many electro-magnetic properties, storing energy and then releasing it, sometimes as ultraviolet energy. Clay can absorb and store many toxic chemicals, heavy metals, and radioactive substances. It can serve as a catalyst for many chemical reactions, and speed them up, in some cases by a factor of 10,000 or more.

In ancient times, clay was packed into wounds or formed into poultices to be applied to burns and abrasions to encourage healing. These earthen packs contained many minerals naturally occurring in the area in which they were found, and gradually certain locales became known for the special healing properties of their clays. Today you can find a variety of purified clays in health food stores, spas, or included in many widely available beauty products. Some examples include French green or rose clay, often used in facial masks, Dead Sea black mud, often used in facial packs or therapeutically for psoriasis treatment, and kaolinite or bentonite clays found in intestinal cleansing products to be taken internally.

Clay masks have a powerful drawing effect, lifting out dirts and oils, clearing dead skin cells from the surface to allow the pores to "breathe," and increasing blood circulation and toning the skin to encourage a healthy glow. A full body treatment will magnify these effects, giving a feeling of calm alertness and invigoration - a great depression reliever! Be careful with stronger clays on sensitive skin, however, as that same drawing effect can leave delicate skin irritated. Be aware, too, that even though some masks come with directions to leave the clay on until it dries, this also can be very irritating to the skin. A treatment can be effective when removed with a warm, moist washcloth while it is still wet to avoid soreness.

Indications for clay treatments can include skin conditions such as eczema, rashes, poison ivy, mosquito bites, or psoriasis; pain relief from arthritis, gout, sciatica or neuritis; reduction of local swelling, or fluid retention related to liver or kidney failure; and toxin absorption in cancer, superficial or deep infections, or heavy metal poisoning. Clay can be used internally to absorb toxins out of the colon as an intestinal cleanser. You can also use the dry powder in shoes to absorb foot sweat and odors.

When mixing your own dry clay (bought at the health food store or even an artist's supply house - red art clay is cheap and effective, although strong), keep in mind that the skin can pass certain molecules into the body, as well as drawing others out. It's best to mix with pure water, cider vinegar, or other clean natural liquid that will support the healing properties of the clay, rather than hinder them. The fine silica dust can irritate the respiratory passages, so use a mask for breathing and goggles to protect eyes from irritation.

For a fun and inexpensive treatment, buy some red art clay at the art supply store (the same stuff they use for making pottery). Take it down to the beach (or in your back yard, although it's rather messy - use a hose for rinsing), mix with sea water, and spread over your whole body. You'll probably want to wear an old bathing suit, since the clay might stain. Leave it on for fifteen or twenty minutes or more, re-applying often to keep the clay moist, then dive into the ocean to rinse. You might want to finish with a salt glow to get all of the clay off. Be sure you are not in a highly populated area, however, to avoid irate beach neighbors, since the clay will redden the water for a brief period of time!

HELIOTHERAPY

Heliotherapy is the use of light for therapeutic purposes. Literally, this means **"sun therapy,"** although modern technology using heliotherapy has been enlarged to include artificially produced light for therapeutic purposes. Sunlight is the basis of all life on earth. It is the energy source that provides us with warmth and light directly. Indirectly it supplies food, clothing, shelter, and energy sources for our everyday existence through plant photosynthesis. We grow plants to eat, feed our livestock and make our clothes, use wood for building and burning, and use fossil fuels for heat, transportation, and factories. Sunlight also plays many vital roles in each organism. Our bodies use sunlight directly on the skin to form vitamin D, which enables us to absorb calcium to strengthen our bones and allow our nerves and muscles to function normally. And daily and seasonal sun cycles, such as the circadian rhythms and solstices, affect other human physiological and psychological states (and help birds know when to fly to warmer climes during winter months!).

Almost all early cultures worshiped the sun and used it as a healing agent - Sol (Rome), Apollo (Greece), Ra (Egypt), Baal (Phoenicia), Woten Odin (Germany), Amaterasu (Japan), and many others bestowed their power upon emperors and kings. **Helios** drove his chariot daily across the sky for the Greeks and was associated with the art of healing. In Greece many people practiced "arenation," using the affects of sun on sand to heal their bodies. Even as recently as the 19th century, physicians were prescribing natural sunlight baths for conditions such as arthritis, rickets, scurvy, swellings, skin problems, and to promote bone growth and healing. Unfortunately, sunlight has gotten a bad reputation in recent years due to the proliferation of sun blindness, skin aging, skin cancer and other diseases, and we have developed a phobia about the sun. We are encouraged to protect ourselves from the sun's rays with sunglasses and sunscreens, which unfortunately screen out the beneficial effects of sunlight as well as the dangerous ones.

Although in heliotherapy we emphasize the therapeutic effects of infrared rays and ultraviolet rays, research is being done now on the importance of **full spectrum light** to health. Studies in the workplace indicate that people are less often depressed and fatigued, more productive with fewer errors, and have fewer illnesses when they are allowed to do their work under lights which most closely approximate natural sunlight. If you're interested in experimenting for yourself, you can buy full-spectrum lamps, or full-spectrum fluorescent bulbs to fit existing lamps (see end of chapter for references). A few things you might want to check for when buying these lamps include making sure the cathodes (ends of the bulb) are shielded with lead-impregnated tape to eliminate dangerous x-ray emissions, converting your system from AC to DC current to reduce flickering and save energy, and using a UV-transmitting diffuser, egg-crate type diffuser, or no diffuser to avoid absorption of the UV range.

The sun's rays vibrate earthward at a rate of 186,000 miles per second. While it is apparent that its rays consist of silvery white light, we have come to know that white light includes violet, indigo, blue, green, yellow, orange, and red, to make up the visible spectrum. The human eye sees less than 1% of the total spectrum. We also know that there are other, invisible rays with properties such as the ability to conduct sound, or penetrate or heat up solid tissues. There are many ways of approaching the phenomenon of light. It has some properties of both particles and waves, although wavelengths, in **angstrom units or nanometers**, are the most common method of measurement. An angstrom unit (A.U. or å) is equivalent to 1/10,000,000th of a millimeter or 1/254,000,000th of an inch, while a nanometer (nm) is 1 billionth of a meter. The different wavelengths are often expressed as an **electromagnetic spectrum**, with the wavelength measured from crest to crest, from 0.0000000000003937 of an inch for cosmic rays up to 545 meters for radio broadcast waves and 3,100 miles (4,990 km) for electric waves from a 60 cycle generator. The visible field ranges from violet (4000 A.U.) thru red (7800 A.U.) Shorter than visible rays are ultraviolet, and longer than visible rays are infrared, since "ultra" and "infra" refer to frequency, or the number of vibrations per second, and not wavelength, which is the distance between successive vibrations of the wave.

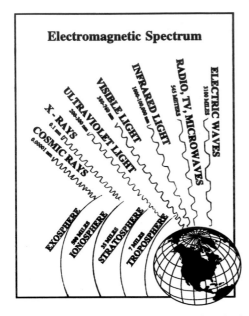

Here is a simple explanation of how different wavelengths are produced. Molecules of both solids and gases are in constant motion. Collision between molecules occurs frequently, which can initiate light waves. This motion and frequency of collision increases rapidly with increases in temperature. At temperatures below 500° C, the energy produced is in the infrared area of the spectrum. At higher temperatures, visible light is also produced, and as it continues to go up, the light becomes whiter until the ultraviolet spectrum is achieved. Our sun has an area called the photosphere which seems to emit a continuous spectrum, with the temperature being 6,000° C. When this continuous spectrum enters the earth's atmosphere, a large part of the UV region is absorbed before it reaches the surface. The much-discussed **ozone layer** is an important atmospheric layer that helps to filter out some of the wavelengths at the ultraviolet end of the spectrum that are harmful in large doses. This ozone layer is damaged by both human technology, such as propellants in aerosol sprays, and natural phenomena. It's interesting to note that the eruptions of Mount St. Helens in 1981 caused more damage to the ozone layer than all of the aerosol spray cans in the history of man.

Note that visible light and the longer infrared rays pass through window glass - in a phenomenon known as the "greenhouse effect," the interior of rooms with windows can become very warm when the sun shines in. Clouds, however, can block infrared rays, as you well know if you've ever been sunbathing on the beach - when a cloud passes in front of the sun, it can get quite chilly! We'll find just the opposite effects with the much shorter ultraviolet rays - glass will block the UV rays, while clouds do not (yes, you can get a sunburn on a cloudy day)! We also find variations in the amount of radiation of both of these wavelengths, depending upon the time of day (strongest at noon), the season (more intensity in the summer months), earth's latitude (stronger effects closer to the equator), and elevation (more rays penetrate at higher elevations, since there is less atmosphere to filter them out). The surrounding environment also has an effect on the amount of rays to which we can be exposed. White surfaces (snow reflects up to 85% of UV rays) and shiny surfaces, for example, reflect many of the rays, while dark and textured surfaces will tend to absorb more.

Infrared Light

In heliotherapy, therapeutic use is made of the infrared and ultraviolet rays. The infrared rays are also known as **"heat rays"** since their primary effect is that of a **local thermal heat treatment**, and thus the effects, contraindications, and uses of infrared therapy would be the same, as is the duration of 20 minutes or more. In therapy, use is made of infrared lamps, applying the same cautions and preparations as for ultraviolet (UV) application with lamps, which will be discussed in the section on UV light following. The distance of the lamp from the area to be treated can be as little as 18 inches. Infrared technology was developed during WWII by the military for "sniper scopes" which magnified the infrared rays radiating from living creatures to allow "seeing in the dark."

Ultraviolet Light (UV)

The major source of UV light, once widely used and natural in origin, is the sun. UV light was first observed in 1801 by Johann Ritter, a German physicist who knew that visible violet light had the ability to reduce silver chloride to silver. When he placed some silver chloride just outside the violet range of a prism-created spectrum, the same reaction occurred. "Black light" is what's known as "near UV" light, just below the visible spectrum. Clinically, UV is administered by artificially produced UV light generators (lamps), at a 90° angle to the bare skin, with goggles to protect the eyes and draping to protect the genitals being very important. The distance of the lamp from the areas to be treated depends on the strength of the lamp, sensitivity of the client, and duration and frequency of the treatment. The usual distance range is 24"- 40," while the dosage is limited to 30 seconds for the first treatment, and further treatments should not be increased by more than 30 seconds per treatment to a maximum of 7 ½ minutes per area (this does not mean you can only stay in the sun for this length of time!). Before a treatment the therapist should take a thorough **history,** check for specific **contraindications, explain** the procedure, **check all parts of the lamp** for stability and electrical integrity, and **drape** body areas not being treated. In the case of **overdose** or electrical shock, **discontinue the treatment (pull the plug) and call a doctor** immediately. In many cases, overexposure symptoms do not show up for several hours, and clients should be made aware of this fact. You might want to test a small skin area for a reaction before doing the treatment, and you'll definitely want to check for medications which might make them more sensitive to UV light.

As mentioned previously, UV light has many effects on the human body, some, in moderation, vital to life, and others, especially with extreme doses, which can be harmful or fatal. Our homeostatic response to UV rays is tanning, where the pigment glands in the skin increase the production of melanin, which causes the skin to darken to limit the amount of UV rays absorbed. The eyes, which have less protection, are susceptible to **"snow blindness,"** a reversible but sometimes damaging inflammation of the superficial cornea of the eye. In extreme doses, especially after extreme sunburns as a child or teenager, skin cells undergo a random mutation of their DNA structure, setting in motion the

---

ABCD method of early detection of melanoma:

A = Asymmetry of mole shape
B = Border irregularities, edges ragged or blurred
C =Color variation in a mole, **changing** color
D = Diameter 6 mm + (pencil eraser size)

Risk Factors for melanoma:

1) Blond or red hair, freckles on upper back
2) Relatives with melanoma
3) Rough red bumps from the sun
4) Three or more blistering sunburns as a child
5) Three or more years at an outdoor summer job
   as a teenager

development of cancerous moles which develop later in life. There are many forms of skin cancer, the most malignant of which being **melanoma**, which is life-threatening if not treated early enough. This cancer of the melanocytes (pigment producing cells) has a very rapid rate of **metastasis**, or spreading, into the lymphatic system and from there to other parts of the body. If you have any of the risk factors and/or notice changes in an existing mole, you should have it checked by a doctor immediately!

On the plus side, though, ultraviolet light striking the skin is vital to stimulate the formation of Vitamin D, a necessity for absorption of calcium from our intestines. Recent studies have indicated that sunlight is perhaps more important than increased intake of calcium for the prevention of osteoporosis, a bone weakening disease which cripples older people, in particular post-menopausal women. And before milk products were irradiated with artificial Vitamin D, **rickets** was an extremely prevalent disease among children, wherein the weight of the child's body actually bowed and malformed the weak bones. Another important function of UV light is mood elevation. It is no accident that Alaska has the highest rate of suicide and alcoholism in the United States, since the limited availability of sunlight in winter months causes people to fall into deep depressions. UV light absorbed regularly over a period of time has been shown to have beneficial effects on the immune system and the body's adaptation to stress, on muscular strength and endurance, resting heart and respiratory rates, and blood sugar and cholesterol levels. Artificial UV generators are commonly used therapeutically to treat babies with jaundice by lowering the toxic bilirubin levels in their bloodstream. Modern technology also makes use of the germicidal effects of UV light to sterilize toothbrushes and other tools. And the pineal gland deep in the brain is directly affected by sunlight passing through the eyes. In the absence of UV rays, the production of melatonin (not the same as melanin in the skin!) by that gland is increased, which in turn inhibits growth and normal sexual maturity. Did you ever wonder why so many animals have babies in

Effects of UV Light

Immediate:
- Vitamin D formation
- Mood elevation
- Tanning, sunburn
- Germicide
- Snow blindness
- Melatonin levels ↓

Long Term:
- Strengthen immunity
- Prevent osteoporosis
- Strengthen muscles
- Increase endurance
- Relieve stress
- Resting heart rate ↓
- Respiratory rate ↓
- Blood sugar levels ↓
- Cholesterol levels ↓
- Bilirubin levels ↓
- Skin cancer
- Wrinkles
- Eye damage

springtime, when the days become longer?

Many skin diseases are greatly helped by exposure to sunlight. Boils, shingles, and decubitus ulcers (bedsores or pressure sores over bony prominences due to lack of circulation) all benefit. Along the Dead Sea coast in the Near East, many retreat centers have been established for the treatment of psoriasis, an incurable skin disease characterized by painful thickened and peeling lesions on the skin surface, which seems to go into remission after bathing in sunlight and the extremely salty Dead Sea. Rheumatoid and osteoarthritis, as well as rickets, are greatly benefited by exposure to UV light, as are many ear, nose and throat problems (earache, nasal congestion, tonsillitis) and respiratory diseases.

There are **contraindications**, however, which go beyond avoiding sunburn and skin cancer. Acute or inflamed skin conditions, such as herpes simplex ("cold sores" - try ice), eczema, and lupus erythematosus, do not respond well to sun exposure. People on medication for high blood pressure or diabetes may find that their drug dosages are thrown off, since UV light tends to lower blood pressure and blood sugar. Cardiac arrhythmia, pulmonary tuberculosis, a high body temperature and certain nervous conditions also contraindicate for UV therapy. And certain medicines, such as sulfa drugs, will intensify the effects of UV light.

UV Indications

- Boils, shingles
- Decubitus ulcers, psoriasis
- Arthritis
- Ear, nose, throat problems
- Respiratory diseases

UV Contraindications

- Sunburn, skin cancer
- Medicines intensifying UV lite
- Herpes simplex, eczema, lupus
- High blood pressure*
- Diabetes*
- Cardiac arrhythmia
- Pulmonary TB
- High body temperature
- Some nervous conditions
- Pregnancy (UV lamp)
*Medicine ineffective, dangerous

Erythema and Burns

The mechanism by which UV light affects the skin is called **erythema**. This refers to an area of skin reddening in response to internal irritation caused by an external influence, such as sunlight or wind. Superficial capillaries dilate and become congested, exhibiting redness (rubor), heat (calor), and sometimes pain (dolor) and swelling (tumor). Erythema can be categorized into **4 degrees**. In the **first degree,** slight rubor results within 6-12 hours after exposure, disappearing within 24 hours. The **second degree** exhibits a slight sunburn, followed by mild peeling and pigmentation in most people. The **third degree**

Comparison of Erythema to Burns:

Degrees of **Erythema**
1st - Slight rubor, disappears in 24 hrs
2nd - Slight sunburn, tanning
3rd - Severe sunburn (1st° burn)
4th - Blisters, tumor, scars (2nd° burn)

Degrees of **Burns** - relative to skin layers
1st - Epidermis only
2nd - Dermis & Epidermis
3rd - Subcutaneous tissues

is a severe sunburn, causing itching and burning, while the epidermis develops blotchy pigmentation (this is comparable to a first degree burn.) The **fourth degree** of erythema is the most intense, causing blister formation, swelling, pain and sometimes scarring. This results from injury to the deeper layer of the skin called the dermis (comparable to a second degree burn). Note that **sunlight cannot cause a third degree burn**, which is the most intense burn, involving damage not only to the epidermis and dermis, but to subcutaneous tissues as well. Often there is no pain in a third degree burn because nerve endings are destroyed, but there is major scarring, requiring skin grafts to prevent debilitating and disfiguring contractures. These burns can be white, tan, brown, black, or cherry red.

Methods to Determine Extent of Burn

Rule of Palms:
- Each palm = 1% surface

Rule of "Nines" -Totals 100%:
- Head front & back = 9%
- Each arm = 9% x 2
- Each leg front = 9% x 2
- Each leg back = 9% x 2
- Torso front = 18%
- Torso back = 18%
- Perineum (genitals) = 1%

Treatment of burns includes ice or cold water applications, sterile dressing application to protect injured tissues from air and infections, replacement of fluids and electrolytes, and use of a Hubbard tank to remove dead tissues, cleanse wounds, and increase circulation and healing. Because blistering burns can cause so much damage to the protective layer of skin covering our body, it is important to figure out how much of the body surface area has been damaged, and how much fluid must be replaced, so homeostasis can be restored (see box).

As we can see, **sunlight in moderation** is necessary to our overall health, but too much can have drastic and deadly effects. We noted earlier that UV light can pass through clouds, so it's best to be careful that we don't over-expose our bodies even on dark days. Remember that the **time** of day, **season** of the year, and the **latitude** and **elevation** of our location will all have an effect upon how much radiation we are exposed to - avoid extensive exposure in the 10:00 am to 2:00 pm time period, especially during the summer in the mountains of Hawaii! UV light can be **reflected upward or sideways** off many surfaces, so don't assume a hat will completely protect you. Some **clothing** will also allow UV rays to penetrate, so you can get a sunburn even while fully dressed, if you're exposed to a lengthy and/or intense dose of sunlight. Certain **medications**, also, can effect how susceptible we are to the sun. Sulfa drugs (antibacterial agents), some diabetes medications, diuretics for high blood pressure, tranquilizers (such as librium), heart medications (quinidine), antibiotics (tetracycline, etc), some antihistamines, and certain soap or cosmetic ingredients, can all cause exaggerated sunburns or rashes.

Sources for Full-Spectrum Fluorescent Lights:

"Vita-Lite"
Duro-Test Corporation
9 Law Drive
Fairfield, NJ 07007
800-289-3876

"Chroma 50"
GE Lighting Product Service
Nela Park
Cleveland, OH 44112
800-626-2000

"Colortone 50"
North American Phillips
200 Franklin Square Drive
Somerset, NJ 08873
800-752-2852

"Design 50"
GTE Products Corporation
US Lighting Division
Danvers, MA 01923
800-225-5483

"Ott Light"
Ott Light Systems, Inc.
306 East Cota Street
Santa Barbara, CA 93101
800-234-3724

APPENDIX A: MUSCLE SORENESS

Causes of Muscle Soreness: If you have exercised regularly or been involved in one or more sports, you have undoubtedly become familiar with muscle soreness; that which you feel immediately following an activity and that which has a delayed onset. **Immediate muscle soreness** is due to a buildup of metabolic by-products such as lactic acid and a lack of sufficient oxygen (ischemia). The cause of **delayed- onset muscle soreness**, which begins 24-72 hours after an activity, is not yet determined. **Muscle soreness is most likely to occur when you perform an activity beyond what your body is accustomed to, when you repetitively use the same muscles for extended periods, when your activity is jerky or bouncy, or when your activity includes eccentric contractions.** There are three theories, each of which has received some support through scientific research. These theories are outlined below:

> 1. **Muscle Damage:** As a result of repetitive contractions, microscopic tears occur within the muscle fibers themselves, causing pain and leading to inflammation, which creates more pain.
>
> 2. **Damage to the Connective Tissue:** Microscopic tears occur in the connective tissues, particularly as a result of eccentric contractions, which are contractions in which the muscle lengthens rather than shortens. Eccentric work is also called negative work, and includes lowering weights with control, running downhill, or landing from a jump.
>
> 3. **Pain/ Ischemia/ Spasm Cycle:** The lack of oxygen and buildup of metabolic by-products causes pain, which causes the muscle to spasm. This further reduces the oxygen available and increases the metabolic by-products, and the vicious cycle continues.

To Relieve Muscle Soreness, Do Things Which Will:

> 1. **Increase blood flow and oxygen to the area** (to facilitate the breakdown of metabolic by-products, and the removal of debris, and to speed nutrients to the cells for healing).
>
> 2. **Relax the muscles** and restore normal length and function.

Each of the following activities acts in both of the above ways: (**The sooner you begin them after your strenuous activity, the better!**)

1. **Stretching:** Stretching should be coordinated, repetitive and not forced (breathe out as you stretch!). Stretch a muscle just until you feel the stretch, then maintain that position until you feel the muscle let go (most stretch comes in the first 10 seconds) OR contract the opposing muscles, & repeat the stretch 10 times, holding no longer than 1-2 seconds each time, relaxing in between. **Bouncing, balancing in extremely stretched positions, or trying to stretch too far will do more harm than good! Stretch gently before & thoroughly after activities** to minimize soreness.

2. **Light Exercise:** Muscles that are not used will become stiff and take longer to become pain-free. Gentle, non-stressful exercise will increase the circulation and relax your muscles. This is the "hair of the dog that bit you" approach!

3. **Massage:** Massage acts much like light exercise or gentle stretching by increasing your circulation, and encouraging the muscles to relax. The difference is that with massage you don't accumulate more metabolic waste products in the muscles to irritate them. The massage therapist can locate and work with those areas of your musculature most in need of attention, encourage venous & lymph flow toward the heart, and discuss ways for you to minimize recurrences.

4. **Cold: Cold water or ice breaks into the pain/ ischemia/ spasm cycle - indirectly by increasing the reflex circulation and directly by interfering with the pain signals (numbing). Ice is also an excellent anti-inflammatory agent, helping to prevent further injury due to ischemia, and will greatly speed healing. **When in doubt whether to use heat or ice, use ice!** NOTE: Don't leave ice on skin for more than 15-20 minutes at a time -- you might get frostbite!

5. **Alternating Hot and Cold: Since the thought of heat often seems more soothing, it is included here, but in combination with cold. Hot water will relax muscles and increase circulation, but it will also increase swelling and inflammation within muscle fibers. Therefore, it is important to alternate with cold and end with cold. This can take the form of a sauna and cool swim, a hot whirlpool and cold plunge, a hot and cold shower, or a hot Epsom salts or cider vinegar bath and ice massage.

**6. <u>Movement in the Pool:</u> Water supports your body weight and makes it easier to work sore muscles. If you are extremely sore, it will be easier for you to use your muscles in the pool -- either walking, stretching, or gently swimming. Many tools are available to enhance water resistance to aid muscle strengthening & circulation, or help you maintain your balance in the water.

7. <u>Aspirin, Ibuprofen, or other Anti-Inflammatory Agents:</u> These help to reduce swelling, and break into the pain/ spasm/ ischemia cycle to promote pain relief and healing. Remember that they may have side effects with prolonged use, or you may be particularly sensitive to one or another, and use them accordingly.

**8. <u>Drink Water, Eat Fruits and Vegetables, Whole Grains, and Low-Fat Dairy Products, Fish or Fowl, & **Sunbathe:</u> Your body needs lots of water to prevent cramping and heal injured tissues, vitamins and minerals (especially calcium, magnesium, zinc, potassium, and vitamins "C," "D," & "E") to heal and maintain healthy tissues, complex carbohydrates and "B" vitamins for energy, and protein to rebuild muscle fibers. UV light is very important for strong, healthy bones & joints, high energy levels, and to relieve stress.

9. <u>Get Plenty of Rest!</u> Also, concentrate on breathing (in and out) during stretch and exercise, as this will aid relaxation.

** Hydrotherapy and heliotherapy applications

APPENDIX B: INJURY PREVENTION

<u>Common Causes of Injury</u> - Many dance & sports injuries are referred to by doctors as "overuse" injuries, actually a combination of overuse, misuse & abuse:

-**Misalignment - muscular imbalance - postural distortion:** Overwork of muscles opposing gravity
-**Faulty technique -** weakness or inflexibility in key muscle groups, substitution of inefficient muscles
-**Poor environment -** hard, slippery or sticky playing surface; excessive heat or cold temperatures; also footwear (or lack thereof) & costumes which inhibit movement, don't protect, etc
-**Poor health habits** - lack of sleep, poor diet, drug use, working beyond limits
-**Emotional**, psychological, family **problems,** eating disorders
-**Excessively high or low body weight**
-**Improper or no warmup & cooldown** exercises/stretches
-**Lack of knowledge** in preventing minor problems from becoming major injuries

<u>Areas of Concern</u>:

-**Weakness/** lack of use of **abdominal muscles -** lower/upper rectus abdominis to stabilize pelvis, prevent lordosis; obliques for trunk rotation - vital in arabesque, extensions, etc; & transverse abdominis - compression of abdominal contents to support low back & relieve pressure on hips, knees, ankles, toes
-**Mis-use or non-use of breath** for nutrition, support & expression
-**Stabilizing muscles balancing movement muscles -** often the emphasis is on turnout of the gesture leg, while turnout & stability of standing leg & torso is neglected
-Tight **hip lateral rotators** (turnout) with weak **medial rotators** (turn in) / Overstretched & weak **adductors** (inner thigh) with tight & weak **abductors** (outer hip) - These can be compounded by **forcing turnout (rotation) at the flexed knee** joint.
-Short **hip flexors** (front hip) w/overstretched **medial hamstrings** (tight lateral hamstrings) & weak **abdominals** w/ tight **low back muscles** leads to lordosis; **slumping or "tucking under"** (overusing gluteus max) leads to back pain & painful "popping" in front of hip.
-Tight & overused ankle **plantarflexors** (foot pointers - back calf) w/weak **dorsiflexors** (front of calf - flexors)
-**Flattened arches,** weak & overstretched ankle supinators (inside of ankle, calf) with tight & overused ankle pronators (outside of ankle & calf) leads to ankle or foot injury, bunions, etc.
-**Shoulders rolling forward (leads to kyphosis),** tight chest muscles with weak

& overstretched upper back & neck muscles, winged scapula (wing bones sticking out); **"forward head,"** tense, rigid **"military neck."**
-**Functional scoliosis** - side to side muscular imbalance in back causing lateral curve w/rotation - always working w/"good side" instead of building up weaker side.

Injury Treatment Sequence:

-For **acute** injury (can take 24-72 hours or more in this phase) w/cardinal signs of swelling, pain, redness, heat & sometimes loss of function - **RICE:** Rest, ice application,* compression wrap, & elevation to slow metabolism, limit swelling & pain & prevent further injury.
-Then treat as **chronic** injury (chronic can also be a gradual deterioration due to misuse) - **Release muscle spasm, increase circulation** to promote healing of tissues - Massage therapy, contrast soaks, whirlpool, ice with stretching, strengthening (cryostretch, cryokinetics).*
-**Stretching** to normal resting length of shortened injured muscles - restore full range of motion, stretch scar tissue to eliminate adhesions that limit range of motion (ROM), gradually increase ROM (lengthen muscles).
-**Rebuild previous strength & endurance** - w/theraband, weights, etc.
-**Increase strength & endurance** to prevent recurrence of injury - w/weights, resistance machines, etc.
-**Increase neuromuscular coordination,** reflexes, proprioception - movement conditioning, balance board.
-Increase **cardiovascular strength & endurance** - repetitive exercise that elevates heart rate to 75% max for 20 minutes or more.
-**Support** all of these with healthy eating habits (a basic vitamin supplement can help), adequate rest, adequate water intake,* strengthening weak stabilizer muscles, stretching tight muscles that limit movement & cause overwork, learning about how your body works & how you can work **with** it!

*Hydrotherapy applications

APPENDIX C: THINGS TO THINK ABOUT

- About 99.5% of all fresh water is in icecaps & glaciers

- The United States uses 450 billion gallons of fresh water every day

- About 75% of water used at home is in the bathroom

- The smallest drip from a leaky faucet can waste over 50 gallons of water a day

- Normal faucet flow is 3-5 gallons a minute, which can be reduced by 50% with a low flow faucet aerator attached - save 280 gallons a month!

- Keep drains clean with a handful of baking soda & ½ cup vinegar left in drain for 1 minute, then rinsed down with hot water

- You can save up to 9 gallons every time you brush teeth by shutting off water

- Save 14 gallons a shave by filling up the sink, instead of letting the water run

- In 6 months a leaky toilet can waste 45,000 gallons of water

- Washing machines use 32-49 gallons of water each cycle (14% total in home)

- ½ gallon of water cooks a pot of macaroni, a gallon is used to wash the pot!

- A trigger nozzle on the hose can save 20+ gallons of water each car wash

- Watering lawns in the morning saves water evaporating in hot sunlight

- It takes 100X more water to produce a pound of meat than a pound of wheat!

- 100 gallons of water used to produce a pat of butter

- 408 gallons of water used to produce a serving of chicken

- 2,607 gallons of water used to produce a steak!

GLOSSARY

Archimedes' Principle: Refers to the buoyant effect of a liquid. An immersed body is buoyed up by a force equal to the weight of the liquid displaced or, in other words, the apparent weightlessness of an immersed body is equal to the weight of the fluid displaced.

Basal Metabolic Rate (BMR): The energy required to keep a resting body functional. The rate or speed of metabolism (calories burned per body surface area per hour) is measured when a person is awake but resting and hasn't eaten in 12 hours. It includes the energy requirements for heartbeat, muscle tone, growth, & other cell activity. Fever increases the BMR 7% per degree increase in body temperature. Fasting slows the BMR.

Circulatory Whip: **Contrast baths** or repeated alternating hot and cold applications (perhaps 3 minutes hot, 1 minute cold) causing alternating fluid derivation and retrostasis.

Conduction: Transfer of heat by contact of one heated object or substance with another object (the method most used in hydrotherapy).

Contraindication: Conditions in which it would be inadvisable to use certain treatments. Contraindications are not necessarily absolute - you might be successful if you modify a treatment according to the person's needs. Peripheral vascular disease is **contraindicated** for thermal therapies.

Convection: Transfer of heat by moving currents of heated liquids or gases (radiators, hot air furnace).

Conversion: Generation of heat by passage of some form of energy through a substance or tissue (ultrasound, diathermy).

Derivation: The act of drawing blood from a distant, internal part due to applications of heat over a fairly large bodily surface area. Dilation of blood vessels of the skin draws fluid towards that area and out of distant or deeper tissues.

Effect: What happens in our bodies as a result of therapeutic measures. Hyperemia is an **effect** of heat application.

Erythema: Skin reddening in response to internal irritation, caused by an external influence, such as ultraviolet light or wind. There are 4 degrees - **1st**: slight rubor disappearing within 24 hours; **2nd**: slight burn followed by tanning or peeling; **3rd**: severe burn with itching, burning and blotchy pigmentation; and **4th**: the most severe, with blister formation, swelling, pain, and sometimes scarring.

Full-Spectrum Light: Research is being done into the importance to our health of not only infrared and ultraviolet light waves, but the full visible spectrum and other electromagnetic waves that normally reach us from the sun (most of the more powerful and dangerous wavelengths are filtered out as they pass through Earth's atmosphere). Glass and brick limit many wavelengths from reaching our eyes or skin, and this may have unhealthful side effects.

Heliotherapy may literally be defined as the use of sunlight for therapeutic purposes, but more broadly as the use of light in therapy. Wavelengths most commonly used include infrared and ultraviolet, but research into the importance to our health of full-spectrum light is presently underway.

Homeostasis: Greek "homoios" (same), "stasis" (standing or staying) - Refers to a state of equilibrium. A narrow range where bodily functions and fluids are maintained so as to support life. A **constancy of the cells' fluid environment** (including extracellular fluid) with regard to **volume, temperature, & chemical content**. If it varies too much the cell or organism cannot function normally and thus may die.

Hydrodynamic Force: Also known as **water resistance**, this is related to the speed of movement, as well as the size & form of the object moving through water. Streamlined objects can move through water with less resistance than blunt shaped objects of the same size, while smaller objects encounter less resistance than larger ones.

Hydrotherapy may be defined as the therapeutic use of water at varying temperatures (including ice, liquid, or steam) and applied by various means, externally over the whole body or any part, or taken internally, to heal sickness and injury and to restore health. The use of hot or cold water in full or partial baths, whirlpools, or body wraps; the steam heat of a Russian bath; seawater or mineral waters for drinking or bathing; water to cleanse the bowel in a colonic; or ice used for ice massage or packed over a sprained ankle to stop the swelling are all examples of hydrotherapy.

Hydrostatic Effect: The shifting of fluid (blood, lymph, intra- & extra-cellular fluid) from one part of the body to another.   Fluids cannot be compressed, as gases can be, so pressure applied forces those fluids to move into another area.

Hydrostatic Pressure deals with equilibrium and exertion of force upon a surface by fluids. This is increased by greater depth and density of a body of water, just as atmospheric pressure increases as one moves from higher atmospheric levels closer to sea level.

Hyperemia: Excess blood flow in an area, due to vasodilation, which results in local temperature elevation and exhibits redness (rubor).

Indication: Situation or condition where a treatment would be beneficial. UV therapy would be **indicated** for babies with jaundice.

Inflammation symptoms: Inflammation is the body's reaction to infection, tissue damage, etc. The cardinal signs include **rubor** (redness or hyperemia), **tumor** (edema or swelling), **dolor** (pain), **calor** (heat), and **loss of function** in the tissues.

Infrared Light: Light waves of the electromagnetic spectrum that are longer than, and with a frequency lower than, visible light. Nicknamed "heat rays."

Ischemia: No blood circulation in an area means no wastes are taken out, and no nutrients are brought in, leaving the tissues irritated and often painful.

Latent Heat of Vaporization: 540 Calories of heat **required** to vaporize a gram of water. This causes the cooling effect of perspiration. 540 Calories of heat **released** when vapor is turned into liquid. This causes steam burns from vapor condensation on the skin.

Latent Heat of Fusion: 80 Calories of heat **are released** when water is changed from a liquid to a solid. 80 Calories of heat **are required** to melt a gram of ice. This makes ice an effective cooling and refrigerating agent.

Melanoma: A particularly malignant type of skin cancer, located in the melanocytes, or pigment-producing cells. This cancer spreads quickly into the lymphatic system, and from there into other tissues of the body. The **ABCD method** has been develop for recognizing potentially fatal melanomas: Asymmetry of mole shape, Border irregularities of a mole, Color variation within a mole, Diameter of a mole that is greater than 6 mm.

Metabolism: The ability of organisms to assimilate food or energy at a chemical level, and use it to perform vital life functions, such as growth, movement, waste removal, etc.

Negative Feedback: Any deviation from normal is resisted. Example: With low blood pressure, the heart rate is fast - the brain signals the pre-capillary sphincters to close off to send more blood back to the heart, then heart is fuller, beats with more force, and more slowly. In the opposite case, when a person has higher blood pressure, capillaries are already closed off or vessels are narrowed, diminishing the total reservoir area for fluid blood, so the negative feedback mechanism would relax the precapillary sphincters and allow the blood to spread farther out thru the system . Less blood would then pass through the heart with each beat, so it would beat with less force.

Pain-Spasm-Ischemia-Pain Cycle: When the body is injured, pain sensors initiate a feedback loop that causes the body to react by "splinting," contracting muscles around an injured joint, and shunting blood flow into the area to prevent further injury. Muscle spasm, swelling, and activated pain sensors result in ischemia, or limited circulation, which causes metabolic waste products and injured tissue to remain in the area, irritating the tissues. This maintains activation of the feedback loop, resulting in more pain sensation, more spasm and swelling, less circulation, increased pain, more spasm and swelling, etc. Therapeutic measures designed to disrupt the cycle can be very effective: ice to control swelling and numb pain, compression or splints and elevation to limit swelling, aspirin, ibuprofen, or other anti-inflammatories to limit pain and swelling, etc. Local circulation will then resume, bringing in nutrients and oxygen, and removing waste products, so that the injury can heal.

Physiological effects of hydrotherapeutic procedures include **thermal** (temperature above or below body norms), **mechanical** (impact of water upon skin surface), and **chemical** (water taken internally).

Reaction: The response of the body to a brief hot or cold stimulus. The heat regulating mechanisms of the body endeavor to maintain thermal and circulatory homeostasis, thru negative feedback mechanisms. There are three phases: **thermic, circulatory, and nervous**.

Reflex (Consensual) Effects: A sufficiently intense local application of heat or cold to the skin surface not only affects the immediate skin area, but exerts an influence thru the autonomic nervous system upon deeper tissues. In general, the skin over an organ is in reflex relationship to it. When a painful stimulus occurs in internal organs, which have fewer pain-sensing nerve endings, pain is felt in the skin and muscle overlying the organs, which have many more sensory nerve endings. Likewise, applying a hot or cold stimulus to the skin will have a reflex effect on the organ. The three kinds of reflex effects: **vasomotor** (circulatory vessels), **visceromotor** (smooth muscle of organs), **secretory** (glandular).

Retrostasis: The opposite of derivation. Characterized by the production of internal congestion brought about by cold applications over the skin. Constriction of blood vessels of the skin drives fluids deeper and towards more distant areas.

Spa: A health resort possessing a source of mineral water, originally named for the town of Spa, Belgium. Broader definition includes health resorts lacking mineral water source.

Specific Gravity: Refers to the ratio of weight of a given volume of a substance to that of an equal volume of water. Water has a specific gravity of "1" and is used as the basis of comparison. Anything with a specific gravity of less than 1 will float, and anything greater will sink in water.

Thermal: Relating to temperature. Thermal physiological effects of treatments relate to applications above or below normal body temperature.

Tonic Treatment: A treatment that "tones up" the body. Cold treatments are referred to as tonic treatments, since cold increases muscular and vascular tone. Often heat treatments are followed by a brief cold influence to prevent excessive heat loss through peripheral vasodilation, thus maintaining the body's homeostatic balance.

Ultraviolet Light (UV): Light waves of the electromagnetic spectrum that are shorter, and with a frequency higher than visible light. Encompasses near UV, or "black light," UVA and UVB, and perhaps others.

Vasomotor reflexes: Include **vasoconstriction** (contraction of smooth muscle to narrow vessel walls) and **vasodilation** (relaxation to widen the vessels).

Viscosity: The cohesive property of a medium, or thickness - this is the property of a fluid that resists forces causing it to flow. Mineral waters are more viscous than plain water, thus giving more resistance to movement through them.

BIBLIOGRAPHY

Abehsera, Michel. The Healing Clay. New York: Carol Publishing Group, 1990.

Asimov, Isaac. The Human Body - Its Structure and Operation. New York: The New American Library, Inc., 1963.

Boxer, A. and Back, P. The Herb Book. New York: WH Smith Publishers, Inc., 1989.

Boyle, W and Saine, A. Lectures in Naturopathic Hydrotherapy. East Palestine, OH: Buckeye Naturopathic Press, 1991.

Castleman, Michael. The Healing Herbs. Emmaus, PA: Rodale Press, 1991.

Chaitow, L. The Book of Pain Relief. London: HarperCollins Publishers, 1993.

Chaitow, L. Water Therapy. London: HarperCollins Publishers, 1994.

Duggan, J. and S. Edgar Cayce's Massage, Hydrotherapy & Healing Oils. Virginia Beach: Home Health Products, Inc., 1989.

Kotzsch, R. "Natural Healing With Water." East-West Journal: 18:1, pp. 33-40, January, 1988.

Hole, J. W., Jr. Human Anatomy and Physiology. Dubuque, Iowa: Wm C. Brown Publishers, 1984.

Kellogg, J. H. Rational Hydrotherapy. Philadelphia: F. A. Davis Co., 1903.

Kime, Z. Sunlight. Penryn, CA: World Health Publications, 1980.

Kneipp, Sebastian. My Water Cure. Joseph Koesel, Publisher, Kempten, Bavaria, 1897. Reprinted by Health Research, Hokelumne Hill, CA, 1972.

° Vierville, J. P. "Der Wasser Kur (The Water Course) Hydrotherapy: Washes, Wraps, Packs and Herbs - Father Sebastian Kneipp and a Hundred Year Health Care Tradition." Massage Therapy Journal: 30:1, pp. 68-76, Winter, 1991.

Perrenoud, A. "Hydrotherapy in the Swiss Alps - the Old and the New."
Massage Therapy Journal: 29:3, pp. 36-40, 42-48, Summer, 1990.

Mayell, M., and editors of Natural Health Magazine. The Natural Health First
Aid Guide. New York: Simon & Schuster Inc., 1994.

Moor, F. B.,Peterson, S. C., Manwell, E. M., Noble, M. C., and Muench, G.
Manual of Hydrotherapy and Massage. Boise, Idaho: Pacific Press Publishing
Association, 1964.

Rodale's Illustrated Encyclopedia of Herbs. Edited by Kowalchik, C. and Hylton,
W. H. Emmaus, PA: Rodale Press, Inc., 1987.

Seeley, R. R., Stephens, T. D., and Tate, P. Anatomy and Physiology. St.
Louis, MO: Mosby-Year Book, Inc., 1992 (second edition).

Tarbuck, E. J., & Lutgens, F. K. Earth Science. Columbus, OH: CE Merrill
Co., 1976.

The Earth's Workshop. 50 Simple Things You Can Do To Save The Earth.
Berkeley: Earthworks Press, 1989.

The Random House Encyclopedia. Edited by Mitchell, J. and Stein, J., New
York: Random House, Inc., 1977, pp 740-749, 758-759, 1526-1527.

Thibodeau, G. A. Anatomy and Physiology. St. Louis, MO: Times
Mirror/Mosby College Publishing, 1987.

Thrash, Agatha and Calvin, M. D. Home Remedies: Hydrotherapy, Massage,
Charcoal, and Other Simple Treatments. Seale, Alabama: Thrash Publications,
1981.

INDEX